The Child Surveillance Handbook

SECOND EDITION

The Child Surveillance Handbook

SECOND EDITION

David Hall, FRCPCH

Peter Hill, FRCPsych

David Elliman, FRCPCH

Radcliffe Medical Press

© 1999 Radcliffe Medical Press Ltd
18 Marcham Road, Abingdon, Oxon OX14 1AA, UK

First edition 1990
Reprinted 1991
Reprinted 1992 (twice)
Reprinted 1993
Second edition 1994
Reprinted 1996 (twice)
Revised edition 1999

British Library Cataloguing in Publication Data
A catalogue record for this book is available from the British Library.

ISBN 1 870905 24 5

Typeset by Advance Typesetting Ltd, Oxon
Printed in Great Britain by Redwood Books, Trowbridge, Wilts

CONTENTS

CHAPTER 6   BIRTH TO 8 WEEKS

THE AUTHORS

David M. B. Hall, FRCP, FRCPCH, Professor of Community Paediatrics, Sheffield Children's Hospital, Sheffield

Peter Hill, FRCP, FRCPsych, FRCPCH, Professor of Child and Adolescent Psychiatry, St George's Hospital and Medical School, London

David Elliman, FRCP, FRCPCH, Consultant and Honorary Senior Lecturer in Community Child Health, St George's Hospital and Medical School, London

WITH CONTRIBUTIONS FROM

C. Bungay, MCSP, Superintendent Physiotherapist, Child Development Centre, St George's Hospital, London

S. Fonseca, MB, BS, MSc, Senior Medical Officer in Audiology, St George's Hospital, London

C. Cullingham, BSc, SRD Cert H Ed, Chief Community Dietitian, Wandsworth Community Health Trust, London

J. Hayden, FRCGP, Regional Adviser in General Practice, Manchester

A. Maclean, BSc, SRD, Paediatric Dietitian, St George's Hospital, London

J. Pearson, SRD, Community Dietitian, Nottingham Health Authority

AND THE ASSISTANCE OF

G. Baird, FRCP, Consultant Paediatrician, Guy's Hospital, London

P. Calvert, FRCS, Consultant Orthopaedic Surgeon, St George's Hospital, London

A. Duizend, SRN (Aust.), HV Cert., Health Visitor and Field Work Teacher, Wandsworth Health Authority, London

A. Elliman, MB, BS, SCMO Adult Medical Services, Croydon Community Health

J. E. Gallagher, BDS (QUB), FDS, RCS (Eng), DDPH, MSc, Lecturer in Dental Public Health, King's College School of Medicine and Dentistry, London

E. Gordon, FRCS, Consultant Urologist, St George's Hospital, London

A. Williams, DPhil, FRCP, FRCPCH, Consultant and Senior Lecturer in Paediatrics, St George's Hospital, London

PREFACE

This book is not intended to be a complete textbook of paediatrics. It is designed for primary care staff who are embarking on child health surveillance and who are faced with clinical problems which in the past were more commonly managed in community child health clinics. This new edition has been revised and updated, and includes much new material.

This handbook deals with child development and behaviour in the preschool years; routine checks at specified ages; immunization, nutrition, accident prevention, and child abuse; and a variety of common clinical problems. It will be useful for all doctors, health visitors and other professional staff in primary care teams.

Details of equipment mentioned in this book, including the Baby Check, can be obtained by sending a large stamped addressed envelope to:

Child Growth Foundation
2 Mayfield Avenue
London W4 1PW

David Hall

HOW TO USE THIS BOOK

Do not try to read this book from cover to cover! It is intended to be both a practical manual, to be kept at hand when you are working in a clinic or in the home, and a reference book which can be consulted for guidance on clinical problems.

It is divided into two sections. The first deals with the aims of child health promotion, and in particular with various aspects of prevention. The second describes normal and abnormal development and behaviour, and outlines the points to be checked at each age.

We suggest the following approach.

Firstly, **look at the diagram** (Figure 1.1) on p. 4 which explains how the book is organized, and note the contents.

Then **browse** through the various sections, and decide which of the material is relevant to you and to each member of the primary care team. Some chapters may well be irrelevant in your particular District; for example, not all Districts expect their primary care staff to test hearing at the age of 3.

Look at the **section headings** so that you will know what information is available when you are faced with a clinical problem. Also, run your eye down the **index** listings.

Then read the descriptions of the **examinations** to be carried out at each age, or, if these are to be done by another member of the team, pass the book to him/her.

If you intend to offer advice on **behavioural and emotional problems**, study these sections carefully; although the ideas in them are simple, they may not be familiar to all readers and they are best studied **before** you meet a difficult case.

You will notice that the male pronoun has been used to denote the child throughout this book. This apparently sexist policy avoids confusion and can be justified by the fact that most health and development problems are more common in boys.

INTRODUCTION

Child health surveillance is a programme of care initiated and provided by professionals, with the aim of preventing illness and promoting good health and development. The precise content of the programme has been debated for years, but the Joint Working Party on Child Health Surveillance, consisting of paediatricians, GPs, health visitors and nurses, recently published a consensus report on the subject, under the title *Health for all Children*.[1]

Traditionally, preventive health care for children has been provided by a separate division of the NHS, the Community Child Health Services (CCHS). However, since the health and developmental problems of young children are intimately related to family circumstances, there is every reason for this programme to be regarded as part of family medicine. The new GP Contract offers a payment for those GPs who wish to undertake this work in their practices. The purpose of this book is to describe both the practical implications and the clinical skills required by those GPs who plan to offer this service.

There are many definitions of Child Health Surveillance, but some authors have suggested that surveillance is essentially concerned with the early detection of disorders, that is, with **secondary** prevention, rather than with **primary** prevention. In this book, we have tried to distinguish between the various approaches to the **promotion** of child health and although we have described some of the methods of early detection in detail, we have also stressed the importance of primary prevention and of working with parents as the most effective means of helping children.

The policies and methods described in the handbook are likely to be accepted by many but not all Health Authorities. Where there is still disagreement as to the most appropriate policy on a particular matter, this is stated clearly and the various options are explained.

[1] Hall, DMB (ed.) (1991) *Health for all Children*. Oxford University Press, Oxford.

PART 1

Health promotion

CHAPTER 1

Child health promotion

Contents

The aims of the programme
Child health promotion programmes
    The inverse care law
Health education—the art of giving advice

The aims of the programme

The aims are:

1 The promotion of optimal health and development.
2 The prevention of illness, accidents, child abuse.
3 The recognition and, if possible, elimination of potential problems affecting development, behaviour and education.
4 The early detection of abnormality, in order to offer investigation and treatment.

In this book, we will use the terminology summarized in Figure 1.1. The unifying concept is 'Health Promotion'. The prevention of disease is only one aspect of health promotion, although it is the area of professional activity which has required the largest share of the available resources. Surveillance has been defined by several authors as being concerned essentially with **secondary prevention by early detection.** It is a term which disturbs some people because of the implication that child health depends on the constant vigilance of, and supervision by, health professionals.

Child health promotion programmes

Child health programmes must be flexible and must meet the needs of the individual child and family. This means that the amount of time devoted to a particular family must be determined by the primary care team. Some families will only

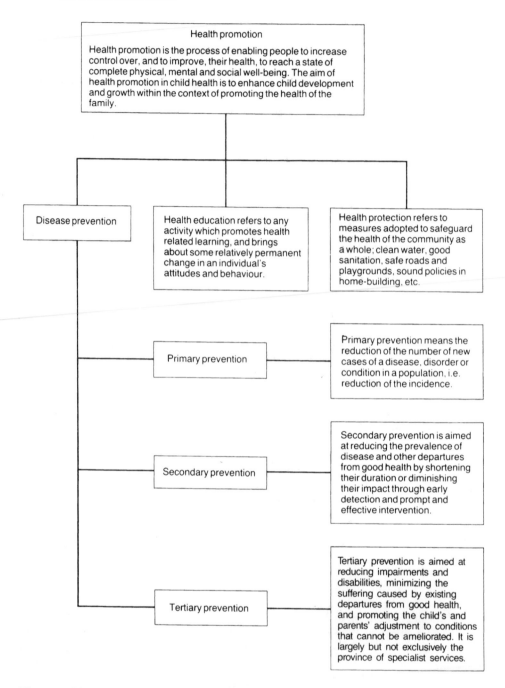

Figure 1.1. Diagram to show organization of the contents of this book.

need to be contacted for specified health checks and can be relied on to contact their doctor or health visitor whenever there is a problem. Others will need intensive professional support.

Immunization and a limited number of health checks are necessary for all children. This manual suggests ages at which these checks should be done, but in reality immunizations and checks are often done on an opportunistic basis; so long as children are not missed and proper records are kept, this is acceptable and indeed unavoidable.

The inverse care law

Middle class families make the best use of Child Health Surveillance (CHS) and expect competent and detailed assessment of any potential problem. The families whose children have the most problems make the least effective use of services. These 'special' families (in most practices, a small minority) need more support and care from the health team. They need advice on all aspects of child care. Without help, they would fail to respond even to quite severe developmental or behavioural problems. It is important to recognize these families and target resources towards them, but it does not make sense to organize the services on the assumption that *all* families have such problems.

The following might be regarded as **priority groups**:

- Very young or unsupported parents, particularly with their first baby.
- Parents of limited intelligence and education.
- Parents thought to be at particular risk of abusing their children.
- Parents who are socially isolated due to personality factors, psychiatric problems, or linguistic and cultural barriers.
- Families living in extreme poverty or temporary accommodation.
- High-achieving parents with extremely high personal standards for themselves as parents.

The medical care of such families is difficult and often needs to be shared with other community services. The role of the health professional is to be a friend and adviser of the parent(s)—the relationship should be established on equal terms, rather than with the professional in the dominant role. The aim is not to change the parent but to enable them to develop as an individual, to increase their confidence and their own abilities in child rearing, and to enable them to make appropriate decisions about their children's health. (See, for example, papers by Dr W. Barker, Early Child Development Unit, University of Bristol, 22 Berkeley Square, Bristol.)

Health education—the art of giving advice

Health education is a potentially powerful means of promoting good health and preventing disease, although it is not easy to measure its effectiveness. This is because the attitudes of individuals and communities are changed only slowly and many different factors play a part.

Child health promotion involves the education of parents about child health, growth and development. It is important to treat the parents as partners in this process, rather than as passive recipients of advice. Simply telling parents to do things is not effective.

Advice is more likely to be acted upon if it is asked for. Try to create the climate in which you are asked for advice.

You are likely to be in one of two positions with respect to the parent(s). One is a **linear hierarchy**; you are telling the parent quite firmly and clearly what to do, there is a well-recognized practice, and you are quite clear what should be done. Advising on how to manage febrile convulsions is an example.

The other position is when you are **acting as a consultant** to the parent(s). You listen to the problem and offer a suggestion as to what might be a sensible course of action, based on your knowledge and experience. You are prepared to discuss and modify your advice if it proves ineffective or unacceptable. You review the outcome jointly with the parent at follow-up. This is the usual model when advising about emotional, behavioural and developmental problems. When applied to parents, it effectively turns the parent into a co-therapist who carries out therapeutic intervention and observes results which they report back to you. It is a shared enterprise.

There are general principles about giving advice:

- It should be seen to be **logical, relevant, and sensitive**. This means that you have to be seen to acquaint yourself with the problem by taking a history, conducting a physical or developmental assessment where relevant, and, if possible, actually witnessing the problematical behaviour for yourself.
- It should be given at **an appropriate time in the child's life**. For example, developmental concepts like 'turn-taking' behaviour, or the process of language acquisition, are interesting to parents if explained in simple terms and demonstrated at the relevant stage in the child's development.
- It must be **practical**. The parents have to be able to carry it out.
- It should be **specific**. Avoid vacuous exhortations such as 'Be more consistent'. If you cannot think how to be specific, ask the parent: 'Suppose I said you ought to be more consistent. How would you put that into practice in real life?'
- **Demonstrate** ways of dealing with behavioural and developmental problems, rather than just describing them. Where necessary, find other parents, nursery nurses or playgroup leaders who can help the parent to learn how to play with and teach a young child.
- Rather than giving advice to stop doing something give **positive advice** to do something different instead. This means saying 'Go out of the room when you feel like shouting at him', rather than 'Stop shouting at him'.
- **Ensure you are understood.** Use specific examples which you have gathered from your experience to illustrate your points. Check the parent understands what you have said ('Do you know what I mean?', 'Can you tell me what you think I've just said?' etc.).
- **Limit the amount** of advice given at any one session. If it is complex, **write it down** and give it to the parents checking that they can read your writing. Record your suggestions in the '**parent-held record**' (p. 110).
- **Try to understand parents' doubts** about the advice given and the reasons for non-compliance.

- **Reassurance is not always reassuring!** Parents who have some concern about their child may be quite prepared to accept that (a) their GP does not know whether there is a problem or not and (b) that the best course of action is to wait and see. They do *not* like to be told that there is nothing wrong or that they are worrying without reason, when they can see themselves that their child has some symptom, sign or anomaly that is not observed in other children of the same age.
- **Use peer groups.** Many young or disadvantaged parents relate more easily to peers in similar social circumstances than to health professionals, who are inevitably more middle class in their orientation. Organizations like Newpin enable parents to share experiences and provide mutual support, which may promote better child rearing and reduce the risks of neglect and abuse.
- **Consider structured programmes.** Many health visitors are enthusiastic about the Bristol Early Child Development Programme, which provides a structured framework for health education on all matters related to the health and development of young children (*see* p. 5 for address).
- **Listen to the parents' concerns.** Health professionals are often too eager to cover the points specified in their Child Health Surveillance programme or their nursing plan, instead of taking note of what is actually worrying the parents.

Readability

If you prepare written information for parents or use literature provided by other organizations, consider how many of your patients will be able to understand it. Readability is increased by (a) short words, short sentences and short paragraphs, (b) a high human interest factor: achieved by the use of personal pronouns, incomplete sentences (e.g. What next? Well, . . .), and references to experiences of individuals and groups and (c) a large clear font, with well spaced text, and sub-headings if the information provided is lengthy. Remember also that a significant proportion of the population is illiterate, or nearly so, and that many people with severe reading problems will go to great lengths to conceal the fact.

Note: Primary and secondary prevention by pre-pregnancy counselling and antenatal screening are not discussed in this book.

Primary prevention

Contents

This section describes four effective areas of primary prevention: sound nutrition and diet, dental prophylaxis; immunization; the prevention of childhood accidents; prevention of emotional and behavioural problems.

Diet and nutrition

Breastfeeding

Breastfeeding should be encouraged as the first choice in infant feeding, but mothers should not be made to feel guilty or inadequate if they elect not to breastfeed their babies. The advantages of breastfeeding should be explained to mothers.

- Breast milk is an ideal and complete source of nutrients for the first 4–6 months of life. It continues to be a valuable source of nutrients even after weaning, as part of a mixed diet, throughout the first year of life.
- Colostrum has a high concentration of immunoglobulins and other substances which are thought to contribute to the infant's gut immune defences, thus safeguarding the infant against infection. These agents are also found in mature human milk, though not in such high concentrations.
- Breast milk is not liable to contamination by pathogenic bacteria.
- It is always available at the correct temperature and concentration; it is convenient and is less expensive than formula.
- It may reduce the incidence of allergic and atopic responses in infants, particularly in families with a history of allergy and atopy, although this is controversial.
- It reduces the chance of hospital admission for gastroenteritis, even in a developed country like the UK.
- There are also benefits for the mother: breastfeeding is, for many mothers, psychologically satisfying; it stimulates uterine involution; it uses energy stores which helps the mother to lose weight; the incidence of pre-menopausal breast cancer may be reduced.

A good start

Maternity units should adopt the code of practice recommended by UNICEF:

UNICEF will designate a hospital as 'Baby Friendly' if it follows the 10 steps to breastfeeding:

1 Have a written breastfeeding policy routinely communicated to all health staff.
2 Train all health staff in skills to implement this policy.
3 Inform all pregnant women about the benefits and management of breast-feeding.
4 Help mothers initiate breastfeeding within half an hour of birth.
5 Show mothers how to breastfeed, and how to maintain lactation, even if they should be separated from their infants.
6 Give newborn infants no food or drink other than breast milk, unless *medically* indicated.
7 Practice rooming-in (allow mothers and infants to remain together) 24 hours a day.

8 Encourage breastfeeding on demand.
9 Give no artificial teats or pacifiers (also called dummies or soothers) to breast-feeding infants.
10 Foster the establishment of breastfeeding support groups and refer mothers to them on discharge from the hospital or clinic.

Primary care staff should be knowledgeable about local services to help breastfeeding mothers: information leaflets, National Childbirth Trust, La Lèche League etc. (*see* box, p. 15).

Mothers should feed on demand and no attempt should be made to impose a routine, at least until lactation is well established and the infant is gaining weight at a satisfactory rate. If the infant seems to be hungry, increased sucking will increase the milk supply sufficiently to meet the infant's needs.

There are considerable variations in the amount of milk taken at each feed and in the time taken to complete each feed. There is no need to insist that the baby sucks from both breasts at each feed.

Breastfed babies gain weight rapidly in the first 8–10 weeks, but the rate of growth may then fall briefly (Figure 2.1); this may worry mothers if they are not aware of the phenomenon.

Problems with breastfeeding

About 65 per cent of mothers commence breastfeeding but only 40 per cent continue for 6 weeks and only 30 per cent for 4 months. Failure to establish or maintain breastfeeding may be due to:

● Errors in feeding technique. The mother should appreciate that the baby takes the whole areola into the mouth to suckle, not just the nipple, and that the 'let down' reflex has to be activated before the milk flows.
● Lack of motivation.

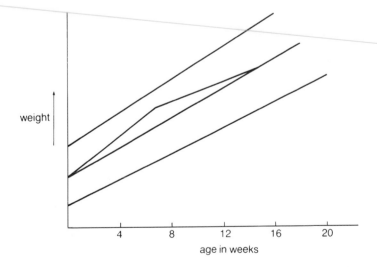

Figure 2.1. The chart illustrates how the rate of growth of a breastfed baby may not be constant during the first few weeks of life.

- Inadequate, confusing and contradictory advice. For example, the mother will become anxious if she does not understand that the milk does not come in for several days after the baby is born.
- Offering complementary feeds in hospital.
- Sceptical family discouraging the mother from persevering. It is particularly important for the father to be positive and supportive about breastfeeding.
- Painful nipples (often due to errors in feeding technique).
- Problems with the baby (ill, handicapped).
- Sleepy baby who does not demand more milk when the supply is insufficient (p. 20).
- Breastfed babies *must* have additional vitamin K (p. 131).
- There is an increased risk of jaundice in breastfed babies (p. 132).

Complementary feeding

This should be avoided; once introduced, it is likely that breastfeeding will be discontinued. The reason usually given for complementary feeding is that the breast milk is inadequate in quantity. To increase supply:

- Increase frequency of feeding.
- Reassure the mother so that she has the confidence to persevere.
- Ensure that her diet and fluid intake are adequate.

If complementary feeding seems unavoidable, the formula feeds should be given after each breastfeed, but only after the baby has sucked for as long as it wishes. Extra feeds given between breastfeeds are more likely to reduce the frequency of demand feeding and ultimately lead to a fall in the supply of breast milk.

It is unfair on both mother and baby to insist on continued breastfeeding if the parents are becoming anxious and distressed and the baby is not thriving.

Additional water is very rarely needed by fully breastfed babies, even in very hot weather.

Fluoride

Fluoride supplements are recommended from the age of 6 months onwards for children at high risk of developing dental caries or for those where the medical condition is such that they are at increased risk of disease on the effects of treatment. Their prescription and appropriate dosage are best recommended by the child's dentist in relation to the individual child's risk of developing tooth decay (dental caries).

Expressed breast milk (EBM)

Mothers may need to express their breast milk if the breasts are very full or uncomfortable; if the baby is small or sick; if she needs to be away from the baby, either for a social function or going back to work. All women should be shown how to carry out manual expression of the breasts or provided with written information, e.g. *Expressing your breast milk*, published by UNICEF.

Breast pumps can be hired from the National Childbirth Trust.

EBM can be stored in a sterile container:

- For up to 24 hours in a domestic fridge.
- Up to 1 week in the ice-making compartment of a fridge.
- Up to 3 months in a deep freezer.

EBM should be defrosted in the fridge for 12 hours, then reheated gently in warm water. Freshly expressed milk should not be added to thawed milk and refrozen.

Diet in lactation

Lactation increases the mother's nutritional requirements; these can be met by eating a healthy varied diet. The mother's appetite is usually the best guide to her energy needs. Low calorie diets should be avoided, because they may affect the nutritional quality of the breast milk. Vegetarians and vegans should ensure an adequate and varied diet with adequate vitamins and minerals, especially calcium and iron; lactating vegans need a source of extra vitamin B_{12}. Some vegan foods are supplemented with B_{12}, e.g. Tastex, Barmene (however, these are high in sodium and are not suitable for infants).

Pregnant and lactating mothers should take a supplement of vitamins A, C and D.

Vitamin supplements

Present Day Practice in Infant Feeding—3rd Report states that DoH vitamin drops should be given from 6 months to 2 years, preferably until 5 years. DoH vitamin drops contain vitamins A, D and C and the dose is 5 drops per day.

Bottle-fed babies

Infant formulas are supplemented with vitamins and minerals and meet accepted standards. Vitamin drops are not required until the infant commences mixed feeding.

Breastfed babies

Breast milk from a well nourished mother meets the nutritional requirements of the infant. Vitamin drops should be given to a breast-fed baby from 4–6 weeks if:

- The mother's diet is poor.
- The mother is eating a restricted diet regimen for any reason.
- The mother is Asian (because of reduced synthesis of vitamin D).

If there is any doubt over the maternal diet, vitamin A, D, C drops should be given—there will be no danger of reaching toxic levels if the 5-drop dose per day is given. Breastfed babies need vitamin K (p. 131).

continued

Vitamin supplements (continued)

Children between 2 and 5 years

Infants' and children's appetites and diets vary considerably over a week and the routine administration of vitamin drops A, D and C will ensure regular adequate intake of these particular vitamins, especially during the winter months.

The child will not receive vitamin excesses if the 5-drop dose once daily is given together with a well-balanced diet. However, it is important that only one vitamin A and D supplement is given.

Vitamin drops should be given by dropper or spoon, not added to drinks or food. The mother may need to be shown how to place the drops in the mouth, rather than at the back of the throat, which may cause inhalation.

Drugs and breastfeeding

Alcohol and caffeine pass into breast milk and should be taken only in limited quantities. For guidance on which drugs are safe while breastfeeding, see the British National Formulary.

The combined oral contraceptive pill may depress milk production, but progestogen-only contraceptives, although measurable in very small amounts in the milk, do not suppress lactation or affect the baby.

It is generally advised that HIV-positive mothers, and those at risk of HIV infection, should not breastfeed; the paediatrician should be consulted in such cases.

Support for breastfeeding mothers

- Ask your health authority for advice about which leaflets and posters are to be used, so that consistent advice can be offered by all health professionals.

- The **National Childbirth Trust** and the **La Lèche League** are support organizations, with national headquarters and local groups in most areas.

- They offer information for *all* mothers and mother-to-mother support, often in liaison with midwives and health visitors. Support starts antenatally, with demonstrations, talks and classes.

- Peer support and encouragement are probably more effective in maintaining breastfeeding than professional advice alone.

- Help is available on a variety of topics, such as positioning at the breast, sore nipples, milk expression and storage, tiredness, jealous siblings, rest and diet.

continued

Support for breastfeeding mothers (continued)

- Mothers find it easier to talk to someone who has had the same experiences; coping alone at home can be difficult but the mother often does not feel that her difficulties justify 'bothering the doctor'.
- Breastfeeding mothers may wish to continue well beyond the child's first birthday. Some mothers feel embarrassed about this and the support organizations help by acknowledging that this can be enjoyable and is perfectly 'normal'.
- Practical help includes hiring breast pumps, supplying nipple shields, fitting and selling a range of maternity bras, access to library material and sale of a range of helpful leaflets.

Addresses:

1. National Childbirth Trust: Alexandra House, Oldham Terrace, Acton, London W3 6NH. Tel: 0181-992-8637.

2. La Lèche League (GB): BM3424, London WC1N 3XX. Tel: 0171-242-1278.

3. Association of Breastfeeding Mothers: PO Box 207, Bridgewater, Somerset TA6 7YT.

4. BFI: 20 Guilford Street, London WC1N 1DZ.

Bottle-feeding

Infants under 6 months of age should not be fed on unmodified cow's milk, because the high sodium and protein load may exceed the kidney's capacity for excretion, resulting in hypernatraemic dehydration. **This is very dangerous and can result in convulsions and permanent brain damage.**

Infant formulas are based on cow's milk or soya protein. The two main proteins of milk are whey and casein. In general, each manufacturer produces one whey-dominant milk and one casein-dominant milk. For example:

- Whey-dominant formulas:
    Premium   – Cow and Gate
    First Milk   – Farley's
    Aptamil   – Milupa
    SMA Gold[1] – SMA Nutrition
- Casein-dominant formulas:
    Plus   – Cow and Gate
    Second Milk – Farley's
    Milumil   – Milupa
    SMA White[1] – SMA Nutrition

Whey-dominant formulas have a whey:casein ratio similar to that of human milk. Casein-dominant formulas have a whey : casein ratio approximately the same as

[1]These no longer contain beef fat derivative, so are suitable for all ethnic groups.

in cow's milk. Whey-dominant formulas *may* be preferable, in that they are more similar in composition to human milk, but there is otherwise no apparent difference between whey- and casein-dominant formulas.

Mothers frequently change formulas because the baby is 'not satisfied', or 'has colic' or has poor weight gain. However, there is little evidence that these manoeuvres help. There is no support for the idea that changing from a whey-based to a casein-based formula will satisfy the baby more easily or that this progression is in any way beneficial. If the baby is not satisfied, the number or quantity of feeds should be increased, or if the baby is 3 months old or more, solid foods should be introduced.

The **volume of feed** required varies. From about 6 weeks babies can monitor their own requirements. The usual requirement is between 150 and 200 ml/kg per day.

Formula milk is nutritionally complete and vitamin supplements are not needed until the baby is weaned on to solids. There is no indication to add sugar to the feeds. Additional boiled water may be offered in hot weather.

Soya infant formula

Soya infant formula has a similar nutritional content to that of a cow's milk-based formula. However, soya milk and milk products do *not* protect against allergic conditions. They should not be recommended indiscriminately for conditions such as 'colic' or for unconfirmed cow's milk intolerance, nor should they be given to premature or low birth weight infants, or babies with impaired renal function. The diagnosis of allergy to the proteins of cow's milk is difficult and should usually be made only by a paediatrician.

Soya infant formulas available are:

Infasoy   – Cow and Gate   Prosobee – Mead Johnson
Isomil   – Abbott   Wysoy   – SMA Nutrition
Ostersoy[2] – Farley's

Only soya milks specifically designed for infant feeding should be used; ordinary soya milk drinks are not suitable as most are lower in energy, calcium, iron and vitamins and should *never* be used in infants of less than 6 months. Soya infant formulas should be continued until at least 1 year of age, and preferably throughout the pre-school years for vegan children. If children on a milk-free diet are consuming ordinary soya milk drinks, they should be calcium-fortified, otherwise a calcium supplement should be recommended. Vitamin drops should also be advised.

There has been recent concern about the aluminium content of soya milk. Mothers worried about this should be told:

- Aluminium is found in varying amounts in all foods.
- Most of the aluminium taken in food is not absorbed.
- The excess is excreted by the kidneys via the urine.
- Once a child is established on a weaning diet, the contribution made by milk—soya milk included—to the total aluminium intake is not excessive.

[2]Ostersoy is the only soya infant formula suitable for vegans because the other formulas contain vitamin D derived from lanolin. All these formulas are free from beef fat so are suitable for Hindus.

Elemental milks

These are lactose-free milks, in which the protein has been hydrolysed so that it is no longer allergenic and is more easily digested. They are nutritionally complete. Elemental milks may be useful for children with lactose intolerance, for instance, following gastroenteritis and in a variety of other conditions. Examples are:

Pepti Junior	– Cow and Gate	Prejomin	– Milupa
Pregestimil	– Mead Johnson	Peptide 0–2	– Scientific Hospital Supplies
Nutramigen	– Mead Johnson		

Cow's milk

Weaning and the Weaning Diet advises that pasteurized whole cow's milk should be used as the main milk drink only after one year of age. It should not be used in the first year as it has two disadvantages:

- Iron is too low at a time when demands are high.
- Vitamins A, C, D and E are all too low.

If unmodified cow's milk is used for older infants the baby must also receive a good mixed diet and DoH vitamin drops. Doorstep milk is microbiologically safe[3] and does not require boiling. Unpasteurized milk is *not* safe and has been associated with many outbreaks of gastroenteritis.

Skimmed milk

Some health-conscious parents are eager to introduce semi-skimmed or even skimmed milk early in the child's life, but there is no evidence that fat restriction in the first 5 years of life reduces the risk of heart disease and it may result in a serious deficiency of energy and failure to thrive. Whole (full-fat) milk should be given at least until 2 years of age and preferably until 5 years. Semi-skimmed milk may be used **after 2 years**, provided that fat and calorie requirements are met from other food sources.

Follow-on milks

Follow-on milks should not be given to infants under 6 months of age, as they have a higher renal solute load than breast milk or ordinary formulas. This increases the risk of hypertonic dehydration with the hazards of convulsions and brain damage.

For infants of 6 months and over, they can be introduced if the parent wishes. They have no advantage over ordinary infant formulas but are preferable to the early introduction of cow's milk.

Follow-on milks include:

Step Up	– Cow and Gate
Follow-on	– Farley's
Progress	– SMA Nutrition

---

[3]Only safe if the cap is intact. Birds pecking the bottle tops can introduce *Campylobacter* infection.

Goat's and ewe's milk

Goat's and ewe's milk are not suitable for children under 6 months and preferably should not be given before 1 year. They are *not* less allergenic than cow's milk.

A goat's milk product is marketed under the name 'Nanny' by Vitacare. There is no known advantage to using this rather than cow's milk formula, it is more expensive than ordinary formulas and there are no data on the growth of infants fed on this diet.

Fresh goat's and ewe's milk is not always pasteurized and is a potential source of infection. It should always be boiled for 2 minutes before using.

If ewe's or goat's milk is used for infant feeding, dietetic advice should be sought.

Preparation of bottle feeds

- The bottles and teats must be washed carefully with a brush. The teats may if necessary be cleaned with salt to remove milk deposits, but it is *essential* to ensure that all traces of salt are removed to avoid the risk of hypernatraemia. Then both bottle and teats must be immersed totally in a sterilizing solution.
- It is acceptable to make up feeds for 24 hours if they are promptly placed in the fridge; but the feed must not be re-warmed and then chilled again for further storage.
- Feeds that are too strong or too weak result from careless preparation. The feed should be prepared with one scoop to 1 fl oz of water (except for 'Nanny'—see above).
- Freshly boiled water should be used. Do not use water that has been repeatedly boiled as this may result in an over-concentration of minerals.

Ready-to-feed milks

Some milks are available in a ready-to-feed form, either in bottles or tetrapaks. They are more expensive than powder milks, but may be useful when travelling or on holiday. Mothers should be careful to avoid contamination when opening tetrapak cartons, by wiping the outside before opening and ensuring that clean scissors are used.

Water softeners

Softened water from proprietary water softeners should not be used for infants because the exchange resin is impregnated with sodium. This exchanges sodium ions for the calcium and magnesium ions in the water and may cause hypernatraemia.

Water filters

Filters reduce the hardness of the water, but the sodium level is not altered. Some water filters use a cartridge containing silver and traces of silver from the cartridge may be found in the filtered water. Whilst no adverse effects have been found from ingestion of traces of silver, water filtered in this way should not be used for infants until its safety has been confirmed. As different water filters use different cartridges, people are advised to check with manufacturers on suitability for infants.

Mineral, spa and spring water

The suitability of these waters depends on the concentration of various electrolytes and minerals. Suitable bottled waters are Evian, Spa, Highland Spring Water,

Volvic and Sainsbury's Natural Scottish Spring. When travelling abroad where the standard of water supply is suspect, parents should use bottled water. The sterility of bottled water cannot be guaranteed and it should always be boiled before use for infants of less than 6 months.

Microwave ovens

Microwave ovens should not be used to heat bottle feeds as heat distribution is uneven; the baby's mouth can be severely burnt by the milk . They are not suitable for the sterilization of feeding equipment.

Weaning

Weaning is a gradual process which begins when breast- or bottle-feeding starts to be replaced by a mixed diet. Disagreements over weaning are a common cause of conflict between mothers and health visitors.

Reasons for weaning

- Milk does not satisfy all the nutritional requirements for a baby from age 6 months onwards.
- To introduce natural progression from sucking to chewing.
- To introduce new tastes and textures to the baby.
- To introduce new skills—use of feeding beaker, cup, cutlery.

Weaning does not commence at the same age or the same weight for all infants, but solids are not usually introduced before 4 months and not later than 6 months.

Food should be offered from a spoon and not added to the milk in the bottle, so that the infant becomes accustomed to spoon-feeding. If the family diet is nutritionally sound, the parents should be encouraged to give the baby family foods; the food can be puréed using a food processor, sieve, or spoon and fork.

Avoiding battles over eating

The first weaning food should be offered in very small quantities, on a plastic spoon. If the baby refuses a food, the plate should simply be removed without any fuss. Force-feeding must never be attempted as it will inevitably lead to severe feeding difficulties. The parent should try to create a relaxed sociable atmosphere and should feed the baby at *his* pace.

Babies have definite likes and dislikes and tend to be conservative about new foods, so these should be introduced slowly and in small quantities.

Difficulties with weaning occur when this advice is ignored. There is often a strong behavioural element to the problem, compounded by friction between husband and wife and by the unwelcome interference of grandparents. These conflicts must be recognized; it is not profitable to deal with the problem simply as a question of nutrition (p. 251).

Poor relationships between the parents and the baby can be associated with feeding battles, meal refusal, feelings of anger and rejection on the part of the parent, non-organic failure to thrive and ultimately even to abuse (*see also* p. 78).

Stages of weaning

Stage 1 (From 4 months): Puréed vegetables, puréed fruit, baby rice, dahl.

Stage 2 (About 5–6 months): Increase variety. Introduce meat, chicken, fish, beans, lentils. Wheat products (bread, wheat cereals, pasta) and egg yolk[4] can be introduced from 6 months.

Stage 3 (About 7–9 months): More variety. Introduce lumpier foods to encourage chewing. Finger foods. As the quantity of solids increases, the amount of milk taken will decrease. Protein from milk will gradually be replaced with meat, fish, eggs, cheese, lentils, beans, cereals. Water, diluted unsweetened fruit juice, or diluted baby juice can replace some of the milk feeds. Introduce drinking from a cup or beaker.

Stage 4 (By 1 year): Minced and chopped foods. Infants will be eating a wide variety of foods such as cereals, fruit, vegetables (including beans and lentils), meat, chicken, fish, dairy products, eggs. Encourage three regular meals and two to three milk drinks (about one pint of milk per day). Additional fluids: water, diluted unsweetened fruit juice. Warn parents about the dangers of nuts and similar foods which can cause choking in babies.

Cultural considerations

Advice given to any ethnic group should take into account their cultural beliefs and foods eaten by the family. Many problems can be avoided if families use their family foods for weaning. Mothers should be taught how to use a sieve, food processor, or electric blender to alter the consistency of the food. They should avoid giving highly spiced foods, e.g. dishes containing ginger, cloves or chilli. Plain baby rice is a suitable base to which mothers can add foods from their own diets. Vegetables and dahls/lentils can be boiled, without the addition of salt.

Manufactured baby foods do not introduce the flavour of traditional family meals to the infant. Furthermore, in some ethnic groups there may be concern about the religious acceptability of these foods; this may severely restrict their choice. In order to avoid using non-halal meat dishes, mothers may purchase only fruit purées. However, there is an increasing variety of manufactured vegetarian baby foods available, so choice need not be restricted to desserts in order to avoid non-halal meat dishes.

By 6–8 months an Asian baby should have tried:

- Fruit, vegetables, dahl, rice
- Cereals—bread, chapatti, wheat cereals
- Semolina
- Natural yoghurt
- Cheese (paneer)
- Lean meat, chicken, liver and fish (if permitted).

If the family is vegetarian, the child should have 1 pint of milk daily and should be offered dahl, cereals and vegetable protein foods. Discourage excess intake of milk (more than 1½ pints daily) as this will depress the appetite at meal times and the diet will become unbalanced.

---

[4]*Eggs*. Because of the problem of salmonella in eggs, it is important to ensure that eggs are well cooked. Raw eggs should not be used.

Vegetarian baby

Definitions

Partial vegetarians. Exclude some but not all animal products, e.g. they may eat poultry or fish.

Lacto-ovo-vegetarians. Exclude all meat, poultry and fish products, but include milk and eggs.

Lacto-vegetarians. Exclude all meat, fish, poultry and egg products, but include milk in the diet.

Vegans. Exclude all animal products including milk. These diets can be nutritionally adequate but careful planning is needed to ensure that serious deficiencies of minerals and vitamins do not occur.

A vegetarian or vegan diet does not preclude normal growth and development, although the more extreme the dietary restriction the greater the risk of poor nutrition.

Protein from animal sources contains all essential amino acids and is of high biological value (HBV), i.e. it is utilized efficiently by the body. Protein from plant sources lacks certain essential amino acids. So that the protein is utilized efficiently, a mixture of these foods should be eaten together to complement each other. For example, pulses and grains can be eaten as dahl and rice, baked beans on toast; pulses and seeds as hummus.

Energy density of many vegetarian foods is low, due to low fat and high fibre content. Infants may have difficulty consuming the necessary volume of food, and growth should be monitored to check that energy intake is adequate.

Parents should be advised to:

- Offer food at least four times a day.
- Include energy-dense food at each meal.

Avoid diluting nutrients in foods by adding too much fluid.

Vitamin B_{12} deficiency can occur in breastfed infants if the maternal diet is not adequate. Vegan mothers who do not take additional vitamin B_{12} have low concentrations of the vitamin in their breast milk. After breastfeeding is discontinued, vegan babies should be given an infant soya formula at least until 1 year of age.

Children's vitamin drops (A, D and C) should be given to breastfed vegetarian infants from 4–6 weeks and to all infants on introduction of weaning foods at least until the age of 2 years, and preferably until 5 years.

It will be difficult for infants to achieve adequate calcium intake unless they are fed sufficient calcium-fortified milk. It is essential that vegetarian infants receive vitamin D supplementation so that Ca^{2+} utilization is maximized.

Other aspects of nutrition

Iron

By 6 months the infant's iron stores are becoming depleted. Iron is included in infant formulas, but unmodified cow's milk does not contain enough for the infant's needs. Iron absorption is increased by vitamin C, but is impaired by the tannins in tea.

Families should be advised on iron-containing foods to include in the infant's diet: liver, red meat, corned beef, iron-fortified cereals (e.g. Weetabix), wholemeal bread, dahl and other pulses (e.g. baked beans), green vegetables.

Non-haem iron, found in cereal foods, is not as well absorbed as haem iron. It may be advantageous to give a source of vitamin C, such as fruit juice, with meals.

Iron deficiency is common in early childhood, particularly in children living in poor circumstances and in those born prematurely. The symptoms are often non-specific, but there is good evidence that iron deficiency does not only cause anaemia but also affects neurological functioning, behaviour and development. These adverse effects are reversed by iron long before there is any rise in haemoglobin level, suggesting that the effect is mediated directly on brain enzymes. Prevention by good diet is preferable to screening but a case can be made for screening infants or toddlers for iron deficiency, particularly in inner city areas. Such a programme is acceptable to and welcomed by parents, particularly when haemoglobinopathy testing is also available (*see* James J *et al*. (1989) *Br Med J*, **299**, 838–40). There should be no hesitation in giving infants a 1-month course of ferrous fumarate or similar iron preparation.

Iron preparations are poisonous in excessive dosage—warn parents to keep them in a safe place.

Sugar

Refined sugar is not required as part of a healthy diet. Addition of sugar to food should be avoided because it contributes to dental decay and may encourage overweight and obesity.

Parents should be advised against putting sugary drinks into feeding bottles or reservoir feeders, especially for the child to hold or take to bed. Such practices result in almost continuous bathing of the teeth enamel with sugars. The use of sweetened dummies should also be avoided. Sugary drinks, many of which are marketed specially for young children, can very quickly lead to severe tooth decay, pain and distress. A general anaesthetic will then be required to remove the damaged teeth. This scenario should be avoided at all costs.

Adding sugar to a feed in order to relieve constipation should not be encour-aged. Fruit juice diluted 50–50, puréed fruit and vegetables will be equally effective in treating constipation. However, over use of fruit juices (many of which contain non-milk extrinsic sugars) can cause decay. In addition, fruit juices are acidic and contribute to 'tooth erosion' (chemical wearing away of the tooth surface). This is very different from tooth decay, but a recognized problem among young children in the UK. Natural fruit juices, if used, should be diluted. Water and milk remain the safest drinks for teeth.

Parents should be encouraged to give children a diet which is low in sugar, both in volume and frequency of sugar intake (Health Education Authority, 1996).

From the start, parents should be encouraged to give children a diet which is low in sugar, both in volume and frequency of sugar intake. Milk and water are the only 'safe' drinks for teeth. However, prolonged bottle feeding should not be encouraged as even lactose contained in milk can also eventually lead to caries. The prolonged administration of sugar-containing medicines can also have a devastating effect on the teeth and sugar-free preparations should be prescribed wherever possible.

Salt

Salt should not be added to food cooked for a baby of less than 6 months because of the risk of hypernatraemia (high blood sodium levels, often in association with dehydration, leading to cerebral damage). When the baby is more than 6 months and is eating family foods, addition of salt in cooking should be restricted to the minimum and no salt added to the baby's food.

Although there has been concern about the role of salt intake in the development of hypertension, there is no definite evidence in support of this hypothesis.

Fibre

An excessive intake of wholegrain cereals and pulses may lead to diarrhoea. Parents should be warned against becoming too obsessed with high fibre diets. High fibre diets are very bulky and have a low energy content per unit volume. The infant's stomach may not be able to deal with the large volumes he needs to yield an adequate energy supply. Parents who persist with such diets may eventually find that their children are failing to thrive and may become frankly malnourished.

Unprocessed bran should not be given to children because it contains phytate which binds with some minerals and inhibits absorption.

Drinks for infants

Often milk intake is reduced when the mother begins to offer alternative drinks, but milk is nutritionally valuable in a child's diet and an intake of 1 pint of milk daily is recommended. However, an excessive intake (over 1½ pints) can depress the appetite for other foods.

Many commercial fruit juices and herbal drinks contain large quantities of carbohydrates in various forms, not necessarily described as 'sugar', and these should be avoided (p. 29).

Offer a parent the following advice:

- Drinks should be offered *after* meals.
- From the age of 6 months drinks can be given from a feeder cup or beaker.
- Take the drink away once the child has drunk all he requires.
- Tea is not encouraged because the tannins in tea impair iron absorption and are a significant factor in causing anaemia.

Common problems

Premature babies

Weaning of premature babies should not be commenced until the baby:

- Is at least 14 weeks old, counting from the time of birth.
- Is at least 46 weeks post-conceptional age.
- Weighs at least 5 kg.
- Has lost the extrusion reflex.

Premature babies should receive iron supplements, 1–2 mg/kg/day to a maximum of 15 mg/day, and multivitamin supplements.

Food 'allergy'

Food allergy and food intolerance have received considerable publicity in recent years. Only a small number of reactions to food are true allergic responses, i.e. involving immune reaction in the body.

Adverse reactions to food can be classified into three areas, (excluding food poisoning which is caused by microbial or chemical contamination of food):

- **Food aversion.** Psychological avoidance of certain foods.
- **Food intolerance.** Abnormal reaction to food, due for example, to a digestive enzyme deficiency.
- **Food allergy.** Abnormal reaction to food involving the immune system.

Food intolerance is commonly suspected by parents and a bewildering variety of complaints have been attributed to 'allergy' to milk, gluten, yeast and many other foods. Only rarely can these 'diagnoses' be confirmed by any scientifically valid procedure, but this fact does not reduce the faith of parents in the power of diet to solve their child's difficulties.

The removal of foods from the diet of a young child has to be carried out with care. If the suspected food is a major source of nutrients, alternatives must be included to make good any deficiency. Advise the parents to obtain a specialist opinion before embarking on such experiments.

Children who have a genuine confirmed food allergy usually become less allergic as they get older and the offending food can often be re-introduced. However, they may occasionally become extremely ill when the food challenge is given, so if the original reaction was severe, this should be done under expert supervision.

Peanut allergy

This is an increasingly common problem. Prevention is important and current advice is as follows:

- Pregnant or lactating mothers from allergic families should avoid nuts in their own diets. The introduction of peanuts and other nuts to the diet of their infants should be delayed until the age of 3 years unless otherwise advised by an expert in the field.

- These precautions are not recommended for non-allergic or non-atopic families. Peanuts of a suitable texture (e.g. smooth peanut butter) can be introduced from 6–8 months of age.
- Whole nuts should not be given to children under 5 due to the risk of choking.
- These restrictions are only of any nutritional consequence if the family is vegetarian or vegan in which case dietetic advice should be obtained.

If a child presents with possible peanut allergy, *either* refer to a paediatrician *or* if you wish to manage the child within the primary care team, ensure that you are following local guidelines. There is still much disagreement about the threshold for prescribing adrenaline. Injectable adrenaline can be life-saving but it is only part of the strategy needed to deal with serious allergic reactions.

Further information:

Patel L, Radivan FS and David TJ (1994) Management of anaphylactic reactions to food. *Archives of Disease in Childhood*. **71**, 370–375.

Anaphylaxis Campaign (parent information, videos etc): 01252 542 029.

Cow's milk protein intolerance

This is a well recognized but uncommon condition and is certainly over-diagnosed. It presents typically at 6–8 weeks of age and the most common symptoms are vomiting, diarrhoea and failure to thrive. Mild cases may present later and the symptoms are varied. Colic without other symptoms is unlikely to be due to cow's milk protein intolerance. Children suspected of having this condition should be referred to a paediatrician to confirm the diagnosis. Dietetic advice should be sought on weaning diets suitable for an infant with cow's milk intolerance, as many commercial baby foods contain milk powder.

Family history of allergic conditions

Allergy to cow's milk is more frequent where there is a family history of allergy. Exclusive breastfeeding *may* have a protective role in preventing food intolerance and mothers should be encouraged to breastfeed for as long as possible, accepting that in some cases the mother may need to restrict or omit cow's milk from *her* diet. If this is done, she will need a calcium supplement. Avoiding gluten until after 6 months may reduce the risk of coeliac disease.

Parents who have genuine concerns based on a strong family history of atopy may be advised to:

- Breastfeed the infant exclusively if possible up until 4 months.
- Commence weaning no later than 6 months.

Foods can be introduced in the following order:

- Baby rice.
- Puréed root vegetables.
- Puréed fruit (non-citrus).
- Other puréed vegetables (peas, beans, lentils).
- Cereals—not wheat until 6 months.
- Lamb, turkey and then other meats.
- Fish—not until 9 months.

- Citrus fruit—not until 9 months.
- Cow's milk/infant formula—cow's milk should not be introduced as a drink until 1 year (although earlier, small quantities may be added to, e.g. cereals), unless breastfeeding has been discontinued or diminished to less than 4 feeds per day, in which case an infant formula will be needed. There is no advantage to choosing a soya formula over ordinary infant formula. Formula milk should be introduced gradually. If an adverse reaction does occur, an elemental formula (for example, Pregestimil or Pepti Junior) should be given.
- Dairy products—not until 10 months. Try yoghurt first, followed by cheese.
- Eggs and nut spreads—not until 12 months.

Foods should be introduced one at a time, so that any untoward reactions can be interpreted.

Gastroenteritis

Babies who develop diarrhoea, with or without vomiting, should stop milk feeds but breastfeeding should be continued. Small amounts of bland solids may be offered if the child is hungry and can tolerate them. Antibiotics should not be given unless there are special indications. Anti-diarrhoea drugs and anti-emetics are potentially hazardous in young children and should not be used. One of the standard glucose and electrolyte mixtures (oral rehydration solutions—'ORS') should be prescribed. The parent gives this by bottle, beaker or, if necessary, by cup and spoon. Although the correct amount can be calculated, in practice the child usually regulates his own intake. Many babies vomit if given several ounces of the solution at once but will tolerate it if it is spooned slowly but continuously into the mouth.

ORS should be used to prevent and treat dehydration. It is not a treatment for the underlying condition. In normally nourished children with mild or moderate dehydration in the Western world, it has recently been shown that the traditional 24-hour period of starvation does not speed the process of recovery. Current advice is that breastfeeding can be continued throughout an episode of diarrhoea. ORS should be given for 3 or 4 hours and other feeds should then be cautiously resumed. If diarrhoea returns when feeding commences, hydration can be maintained with ORS but there is little or no benefit in further starvation.

ORS is highly effective but there are several dangers for the unwary:

- The solution is simply a means of making good the losses of water and electrolytes. The parent should be told the rationale for its use and should appreciate that it is *not* a treatment for the underlying condition. The diarrhoea and vomiting will not necessarily cease at once.
- Diarrhoea and vomiting can be features of illnesses other than gastroenteritis. Every case should be kept under *frequent* review until the baby has recovered. Each year babies die from conditions such as intussusception and appendicitis because the initial symptoms were identical to those of gastroenteritis.
- Most mild cases of gastroenteritis are viral; nevertheless, a stool sample should be sent if diarrhoea persists, or is severe, or is accompanied by blood, in order to identify other organisms including *Campylobacter*, *Salmonella*, *Shigella* and *Cryptosporidium*.
- Gastroenteritis in a healthy child rarely leads to severe dehydration, but this *can* occur; if the baby is becoming too lethargic to take the replacement

solution or is clinically dehydrated, or is acidotic (rapid deep breathing often mistaken for pneumonia) hospitalization should be arranged.

- Do not continue with replacement solution if the symptoms are not improving. The nutritional content is negligible and babies can become undernourished very quickly, perhaps pre-disposing to more serious infections. Do not hesitate to get specialist advice in such cases.
- Monitor growth after a severe episode of gastroenteritis, until it is clear that weight gain is satisfactory.

Assessing dehydration

- **Mild:** minimal physical signs; thirst; dry mouth; slightly sunken eyes; normal pulse and circulation.
- **Moderate:** reduced urine output; raised pulse rate; skin turgor reduced; definitely sunken eyes; depressed fontanelle.
- **Severe:** restless or drowsy; rapid weak pulse; deeply sunken eyes; skin turgor obviously reduced.

NB Combinations of signs vary; do not expect to find all the signs in every case.

- **Acidosis:** indicated by deep 'air-hunger' breathing; sometimes mistaken for pneumonia. Can occur with any degree of dehydration. Needs hospital care.
- **CAUTION:** tender or distended abdomen; bile-stained vomiting; toxic child; bloody diarrhoea; disturbed consciousness; sustained vomiting without diarrhoea.

There may be transient lactose intolerance after severe gastroenteritis. A lactose-free milk can be used in such cases; either a soya milk or preferably an elemental milk such as Pregestimil would be suitable. However, if the symptoms are sufficiently troublesome to merit consideration of such measures, it is probably wise to obtain specialist advice.

Toddler diarrhoea. This is the commonest cause of chronic loose stools in early childhood. It is also known as peas and carrots diarrhoea because the presence of these undigested foods in the stool is often noted by parents. The onset is often difficult to time precisely, though it may follow an episode of gastroenteritis. The motions vary in consistency from day to day and may be accompanied by mucus, but not by blood. Sometimes they are so loose that toilet training is difficult. The crucial diagnostic feature is that the child is absolutely well in every other respect and putting on weight normally. No treatment is necessary. If the symptoms are troublesome, it may help to increase the fat and fibre content of the diet; reduce the amount of fruit juice, especially clear apple juice; control the amount of fluid drunk between meals. Paediatricians often prescribe loperamide, though most parents prefer to use this for outings or special occasions rather than regularly. It is not licensed for children or recommended by the manufacturers for children under 4, but nevertheless it is safe even when used over longer periods. Remind parents to keep it in a safe place as overdose is hazardous.

Vomiting. Vomiting may be associated with diarrhoea in acute gastroenteritis. The sudden onset of vomiting *without* diarrhoea may be due to a simple viral infection, but more serious infections, intestinal disorders and metabolic conditions may also present in this way.

Repeated forceful or 'projectile' vomiting in the first few months of life may be due to pyloric stenosis. Such cases should be referred promptly.

By far the commonest cause of repeated small vomits in an otherwise well baby is possetting or regurgitation, associated with reflux of stomach contents up the oesophagus. This varies from an occasional mouthful of milk with wind to severe reflux leading to growth impairment and/or respiratory disorders.

Possetting, regurgitation and vomiting

To make a diagnosis of uncomplicated regurgitation you need to establish that:

- The baby is well in all other respects.
- The problem is chronic rather than acute.
- The baby is thriving.
- The baby's development is within normal limits.
- There are no respiratory complaints (which might suggest aspiration of stomach contents into the lungs).
- The stools are normal.
- There is no blood in the vomit.

If there is doubt about any of these points, referral is advisable.

Management

- Review the feeding regimen. The baby may be very hungry and feeding too quickly, or the mother may be giving the baby more milk than he can tolerate.
- If the baby is difficult to feed, a home visit to observe feeding and handling may be undertaken by the health visitor, community paediatric nurse or community dietitian.
- The feeds can be thickened using an agent such as Nestargel.
- Introduction of solids often leads to improvement.
- Infant Gaviscon may help.
- Changing the brand of milk formula rarely helps.
- Gradual improvement usually occurs as the baby is weaned.
- Monitor weight gain until you are happy that the baby is thriving.

Additives

The prevalence of intolerance to food additives in the population as a whole is very low, perhaps only 0.03–0.15 per cent. Food additives are added to food:

- To prevent food contamination, increase shelf life, allow a wider variety of food to be available all year round, prevent food poisoning.
- To aid processing, e.g. raising agents in cakes.
- To enhance the colour or flavour of food.
- To replace nutrients lost in processing.

Convenience foods and processed foods are part of our modern diet and life-style, but some additives, such as colouring agents, are not necessary. Children do tend to eat foods with unnecessary additives—fruit squash, fizzy drinks, instant puddings, sweets. The evidence that these additives do any harm is limited, though they may be involved in *some* cases of hyperactivity and migraine. Nevertheless it is understandable that parents should wish to limit the child's intake. Advise them to:

- Use fresh foods.
- Use home-baked dishes instead of bought pies, cakes, packet soups, etc., which have a high number of additives.
- Avoid highly processed foods (additive cocktails).
- Look at the label (the ingredients are given in order of quantity).

'E' numbers. Permitted food additives, other than flavourings, are given a number to aid in labelling. Additives are grouped according to their function:

- E100–199: permitted colours.
- E220–321: preservatives and antioxidants—to keep food fresh.
- E322+: processing aids, e.g. emulsifiers, stabilizers, and aerating, gelling and thickening agents.

Additives without an 'E' prefix are either awaiting approval or have not gained approval in the EC. Some E additives are naturally occurring substances, for example:

- E101 (riboflavin).
- E140 (chlorophyll).
- E170 (chalk).
- E260 (acetic acid).
- E270 (lactic acid).
- E300 (vitamin C).

There is no point in trying to avoid all E numbers.

Hair analysis

Analysis of hair for mineral content is undertaken by certain practitioners, as a measure of the 'mineral composition and deficiencies of the body'. Unfortunately, hair mineral content does not accurately reflect the composition of the body and this procedure has no scientific validity.

Food and poverty

Poor families reduce expenditure on food whenever times are hard. This can have a serious effect on the nutritional status of low income families.

Advice given to individual families must be appropriate to their social circumstances (finance, housing, education, partner support, cooking facilities, cooking skills, ease of access to shops and interest in food preparation). Fuel costs are an important consideration. The gas and electricity boards provide leaflets and information on economic use of fuel during cooking. Emphasis should be placed on eating an adequate diet within the budget and ability of the family. Encourage family meals, as cooking for a family is easier and cheaper than cooking individual meals.

Poverty and poor living conditions are factors linked with the incidence of iron deficiency. Low income families should be told about cheap food sources of iron:

- Cheap cuts of meat have as good an iron content as more expensive cuts.
- Sardines and pilchards have an appreciable iron content.
- Other useful low-cost foods are pulse vegetables and baked beans.
- Dahl and lentils.
- Iron-fortified cereals, e.g. Weetabix.

Vitamin C in the diet helps the body to utilize iron from cereal sources more efficiently. Give DoH vitamin drops A, D, C.

Prevention of dental disease

Introduction

The two main dental diseases are tooth decay (dental caries) and gum disease (periodontal disease). Caries causes most concern in young children and it can be prevented. Unfortunately, many children do not attend a dentist until dental disease is well established. Disease levels vary throughout the country but between a third and a half of the nation's children have experienced caries on entry to school at 5 years of age. An increasing problem is damage to teeth caused by acidic drinks and juices which demineralize teeth causing erosion—thinning of enamel.

Baby teeth are important and should not be neglected. If they are badly decayed, and develop an abscess and/or become painful, the permanent teeth may be damaged. It is important to promote healthy diet and good teeth cleaning from an early age as it is difficult to unlearn bad habits.

Dental caries in children can be prevented as outlined in the Scientific Basis of Dental Health Education (Health Education Authority, 1996) by:

- **diet:** reducing the consumption and especially the frequency of intake of sugar-containing food and drink
- **tooth brushing:** cleaning the teeth thoroughly twice every day with a fluoride toothpaste
- strengthening teeth with **fluoride**
- **dental attendance:** attending every year for an oral examination, and
- avoiding other sources of sugar such as sugar in medicines.

A healthy diet

This is the most important factor in preventing tooth decay. **The volume, and especially the frequency of sugar ingested, should be kept to a minimum. The**

number of times that sugars enter the mouth is the most important factor in determining the rate of decay.

Each time sugar is eaten or drunk, acid is rapidly generated in dental plaque on teeth within seconds and within 1–2 minutes plaque pH has fallen to levels at which enamel dissolution can occur. The return to neutrality can take between 20 minutes and 2 hours. If a high frequency of sugar intake occurs, this will not allow time for the pH to recover and for a large proportion of the day teeth are under attack. Dental caries can quickly develop.

Poor dietary habits include:

- adding sugar to feeds or drinks
- frequent sugary snacks and/or drinks
- the use of sweetened comforters or dinky feeders.

Ideally, sugary foods and drinks should be consumed in conjunction with meal-times as most meals contain some 'hidden' sugar. Sugary snacks are best avoided between meals.

It is important to note that many foods and drinks marketed as 'healthy' or 'for babies and young children' can cause serious damage to teeth because of their high sugar content. Parents should be encouraged to read product labels carefully.

Effective toothbrushing

Toothbrushing *per se* does not prevent dental caries. Its purpose is to remove plaque and keep gums healthy and, to be effective, it must be carried out regularly and thoroughly. Every surface of every tooth needs to be cleaned carefully, paying special attention to the junction between the tooth and gum.

Parents should be encouraged to commence cleaning their child's teeth with a pea-sized amount of a fluoride toothpaste once teeth appear (from approximately 6 months). This can easily be carried out with the parent positioned behind their child, steadying his/her chin with their left hand while brushing with their right hand (vice versa for left-handed people). Children will require assistance to ensure effective toothbrushing up to the age of about 8 years, although they should be encouraged to practice brushing their teeth themselves. Effective tooth cleaning is more important than frequent cleaning. Twice a day is sufficient and it is important that teeth are thoroughly cleaned last thing at night.

Toothbrushing is an important method of applying fluoride to strengthen teeth. Caution in the type and amount of toothpaste used (and swallowed) should be exercised if a child is taking fluoride supplements or the local water supply is fluoridated. In such cases a pea-sized blob of a low fluoride children's toothpaste should be used.

Fluoride

Fluoride strengthens teeth against caries (Murray and Naylor, 1996). If it is present systemically when teeth are forming (from fluoridated water or fluoride supplements), it will be incorporated into the growing teeth. Its presence makes teeth more resistant to acid attack and tooth decay.

Fluoridation of the water supply is the most effective way of getting fluoride to the general public. At a concentration of 1 part per million it can reduce decay by about 50%. This occurs naturally in some areas of the UK and, in other areas, fluoride has been added to bring levels up to the optimum for dental health. Water authorities will be able to provide information on the fluoride levels in local water supplies. The majority of people in the UK do not receive fluoridated water.

After teeth have erupted (appeared in the mouth), they can also benefit from fluoride acting topically on the surface of the teeth from fluoridated water or toothpaste. As many people do not receive fluoridated water, the use of a fluoride toothpaste remains an effective method of strengthening teeth.

Benefit is obtained by taking fluoride supplements from 6 months through to adolescence in areas of low/no water fluoridation. However, compliance with a regimen which requires daily fluoride tablets/drops to be taken for about 15 years has been shown to be a problem, particularly among sections of the population where disease levels are highest. In addition, parents may be rather lax with diet if they feel that their child's teeth are protected by fluoride. Healthy eating should be the main emphasis in preventing tooth decay.

Fluoride supplements can be prescribed by both doctors and dentists. Rather than using a blanket approach to the prescription of fluoride supplements, there is benefit in targeting their use towards individual children with special needs. These include children at high risk of developing dental caries or who have a medical condition where dental disease would prove deleterious to health. Dentists are therefore best able to determine individual and family risk and take the decision about prescribing fluoride supplements and advising on their con-centration based on risk and the local level of water fluoridation, hence the importance of early dental attendance.

If excess fluoride is ingested when teeth are forming, it can cause mottling or staining of teeth, so care must be taken to ensure that this is avoided by making sure that children are not swallowing large amounts of high fluoride toothpaste, particularly if they are receiving fluoridated water or supplements. Only a small pea-sized amount of toothpaste should be used, and parents must supervise brushing up to at least 7 or 8 years (BSPD Policy Document, 1996).

Dental attendance—registering with a dentist

All children are now encouraged to register with a family dentist from birth, as dental care moves from a predominantly treatment-based approach to a preventive one. If a child attends regularly, approximately every year from birth, there is the opportunity for the prevention of dental disease. In addition, children become accustomed to attending a dentist (which can be fun!) and build up trust so that if treatment should be required, it will be easier for the child, parent and dentist. Early detection and simple treatment of dental disease will be pos-sible if dental attendance is regular. Parents experiencing problems in finding an NHS dentist may contact their local health authority or the Community Dental Service for advice and support in finding appropriate care.

Children with other medical problems

Children with frequent illness or chronic disease may require regular medication. Sugary medicines can cause serious tooth decay and sugar-free medicines should be used where possible.

Further reading

1. *Present Day Practice in Infant Feeding—3rd Report.* Reports on Health and Social Subjects, no. 32. HMSO, London.

2. *Successful Breast-feeding* (1988) Royal College of Midwives.

3. Taitz LS and Wardley B (1989) *Handbook of Child Nutrition.* Oxford University Press.

4. David TJ (1993) *Food and Food Additive Intolerance in Childhood.* Blackwell Scientific Publications, Oxford.

5. *Weaning and the Weaning Diet* (Reports on Health and Social Subjects 45) (1994) HMSO, London.

6. Health Education Authority (1996) *The Scientific Basis of Dental Health Education: a policy document (2nd ed).* HEA, London.

7. Murray JJ and Naylor MN (1996) Fluorides and dental caries in children. In: JJ Murray (ed) *Prevention of Oral Disease.* Oxford University Press, Oxford.

8. BSPD (1996) British Society of Paediatric Dentistry: a policy document on fluoride dietary supplements and fluoride toothpastes for children. *International Journal of Paediatric Dentistry.* **6**, 139–142.

Prevention of infectious diseases: (a) immunization

How to achieve high rates of vaccination

*   Give it a **high priority**. Devote time to organizing it within the practice. Give someone overall responsibility for vaccination within the primary care team.

*   Be **enthusiastic** and convince parents that it is important. **Emphasize the benefits**.

*   Be **well informed** and know the true contraindications.

*   **Never say that a child should not receive a vaccination without being absolutely certain that this advice is correct.** There should be very strong grounds for denying a child the benefits of vaccination. If in doubt seek further advice from a community paediatrician, hospital paediatrician or community physician.

*   **Know where to seek further advice locally.**

*   Be **flexible** and vaccinate whenever the opportunity arises.

*   **Liaise** closely with all others involved in vaccination in the District. This includes health visitors, clinic doctors and the District Immunization Co-ordinator.

*   You are probably more likely to be sued for withholding a vaccine than for giving it.

Childhood vaccination

Vaccination of children has been shown not only to be a highly effective form of preventive care, but also to save money. Many vaccines have been in use for decades, but until recently the take-up rates were still, on average, below target figures set by the World Health Organization. Figures show that the average take-up of the triple, polio, Hib and MMR immunizations exceeds 90 per cent.

Introduction

In the 1990 GP Contract two target take-up levels were set. To achieve the lower level of remuneration, an average of 70 per cent of children aged 2 years should have been immunized with the three groups of vaccines—diphtheria, tetanus and polio; pertussis; and MMR (mumps, measles and rubella). To achieve the higher level, 90 per cent need to be immunized. It is obviously important that as many children as possible are immunized, irrespective of these targets.

Immunization schedules vary very slightly from District to District, but that currently recommended by the Department of Health is as follows:

Birth	BCG to those in high risk groups (*see* p. 45). Hepatitis B to those babies whose mothers were Hepatitis B surface antigen-positive during pregnancy.
4 weeks	Hepatitis B (as above)—2nd dose.
8 weeks	Triple vaccine (diphtheria, tetanus and pertussis—DTP), *Haemophilus influenzae* type b (Hib) and oral polio (OPV).*
12 weeks	DTP, Hib and OPV.*
16 weeks	DTP, Hib and OPV.*
26 weeks	Hepatitis B (as above)—3rd dose.
12–18 months	First dose of mumps, measles and rubella (MMR).**
Preschool (3.5–5 years)	Boosters of diphtheria, tetanus and OPV. Second dose of MMR, if not already given.***
10–14 years	BCG, if tuberculin-negative.
School-leaving age (15–18 years)	Boosters of diphtheria, tetanus and OPV. MMR should be given if not already received two doses of a measles containing vaccine.

* DTP and Hib is usually given as a combination injection.
** The first dose of MMR is best given as soon as possible after the first birthday.
*** The second dose of MMR can be given at any time after the first, as long as at least three months have elapsed.

Haemophilus influenzae type b (Hib) vaccine was introduced into the UK on 1st October 1992. Hib is the most important cause of meningitis in children under four years old. Where the vaccine has been introduced, Hib meningitis has almost disappeared entirely. The vaccine is one of the safest in use. Parents must be reminded that the Hib prevents only one of the several types of meningitis.

The intervals between the three doses of primary course of DTP, Hib and polio should not be reduced below the recommendation of 4 weeks. Any further reduction might impair efficacy.

MMR

MMR has been in use in the USA for over 25 years, in some parts of Scandinavia for 15 years and in the UK for 10. Over this period the incidence of measles has fallen dramatically. However, the vaccine has an efficacy of only 90–95%. For this reason all these countries now recommend a two-dose schedule. Recently, concerns have been raised about a possible link between the vaccine and autism and inflammatory bowel disease. An ad hoc meeting of experts organized by the Medical Research Council in March 1998 concluded that 'There is no evidence to indicate any link between MMR vaccination and bowel disease or autism.' This is the view held by all national bodies and the World Health Organisation.

Other vaccines

Other vaccines may need to be given in special circumstances. Hepatitis B vaccine should be given to those at risk by nature of disease-state or contacts. Those with some chronic disorders (severe asthma, cystic fibrosis, bronchopulmonary dysplasia, cyanotic congenital heart disease, etc.) should be given influenza vaccine. It should also be considered in all children with Down's syndrome and those with major neurodevelopmental problems. Tetanus boosters may be needed at the time of injury, depending on the circumstances. Rabies, yellow fever, hepatitis A, typhoid, Japanese encephalitis, tick-borne encephalitis, meningococcal and pneumococcal vaccines may be appropriate in some individuals.

An acellular pertussis vaccine is available on a 'named patient' basis. It may be given where pertussis has been omitted from the primary course or, in some circumstances, where the whole cell vaccine is contraindicated.

Storage of vaccines

Safe storage is essential.

Site of injection

Apart from BCG, and in some circumstances rabies, all injections should be given by intramuscular or deep subcutaneous injection. There is evidence that more superficial subcutaneous injections are likely to give rise to a greater number of significant local reactions. All intramuscular and subcutaneous injections should be given into either the deltoid region of the upper arm or the anterolateral aspect of the thigh. Vaccines should never be given into the buttocks as the efficacy may be reduced and there is a small risk of sciatic nerve damage. Intradermal injections should only be given by those who have had the requisite training and who use this route regularly.

The skin may be cleansed by swabbing, but vigorous attempts at sterilization are not needed. Do not use acetone; it is a serious fire hazard. Alcohol should be allowed to dry before the injection is given, otherwise it hurts, and may inactivate live vaccines.

Audit your vaccine transport and storage

A breakdown in the 'cold chain', the system of keeping vaccines at the correct temperature during transfer from manufacturer to user, is potentially as great a problem in the UK as it is in the Tropics. Vaccines that are incorrectly stored rapidly lose potency.

- One named individual should be responsible for monitoring the refrigerator function, and ensuring that the correct action is taken in the event of a breakdown or error.

- OPV manufactured by Evans Medical should be stored at 0–4°C, whereas other vaccines should be stored at 2–8°C. In practice, this means that vaccine fridges have to be set at 2–4°C.

- An overfull refrigerator will have a wide temperature range within it. It should be filled to 50 per cent of capacity, with spaces between vaccine packages to allow free air circulation.

- The temperature should be monitored with a maximum/minimum thermometer placed in the middle of the refrigerator.

- The refrigerator should be defrosted regularly if it has no automatic defrosting facility. During defrosting the vaccines should be kept in another refrigerator or in a cool bag.

- Food and specimens should not be stored in the same refrigerator as vaccines.

- Reconstituted vaccines must be used within the specified period. Partially used multi-dose vials must be discarded at the end of a session.

- Vaccines should be kept in a cool bag for transport from district pharmacies or between practice premises.

- Whenever vaccines are in use, there should be a tray with resuscitation equipment available. It should include adrenaline 1/1,000, and chlorpheniramine, together with 1 ml syringes, needles and airways.

Contraindications to vaccination

There are very few contraindications to vaccination, but myths abound. The true contraindications are set out below.

- Any vaccination should be postponed for any child who is **acutely unwell** with a fever or systemic upset. A mild illness without these features can be ignored. As soon as the child is well the vaccination should be given. Treatment with antibiotics is not, in itself, a contraindication.
- Children who are known to have had an **anaphylactic response to a constituent of a vaccine** should receive that vaccine only under hospital supervision, if at all. Minor allergic reactions to eggs or antibiotics are not relevant.
- Children who are **immunocompromised**, whether due to disease or treatment, or are **HIV-positive**, should be referred to their consultant for advice.

It should not be assumed that vaccination is to be postponed but it may often be overlooked.

- **Household contacts of individuals who are immunosuppressed** should be given inactivated polio vaccine (IPV) rather than the oral vaccine (OPV) as the latter is transmissible. Many areas make the same recommendations in respect of HIV-positive individuals.
- Pertussis vaccine should not be given to children who have had a **severe local or systemic reaction to a previous dose**. A severe local reaction is defined as 'an extensive area of redness and swelling which becomes indurated and involves most of the anterolateral surface of the thigh or a major part of the circumference of the upper arm'.

  A severe general reaction includes any of the following:

  - A fever equal to or greater than 39.5°C within 48 hours of injection.
  - Anaphylaxis.
  - Bronchospasm.
  - Laryngeal oedema.
  - Generalized collapse.
  - Prolonged unresponsiveness.
  - Prolonged inconsolable screaming.
  - Convulsions occurring within 72 hours.

Treatment of acute anaphylaxis

Anaphylaxis is very rare. Most staff will never see a true case, so occasional *rehearsal* of the management is a good idea.

Diagnosis

- Pallor, limpness and transient apnoea are the most common signs in children.
- Upper airway obstruction: hoarseness and stridor as a result of angio-oedema involving the hypopharynx, epiglottis and larynx.
- Lower airways obstruction: subjective feelings of retrosternal tightness and dyspnoea with audible expiratory wheeze from bronchospasm.
- Cardiovascular: sinus tachycardia, profound hypotension in association with tachycardia; severe bradycardia.
- Skin: characteristic rapid development of urticarial lesions—circumscribed, intensely itchy weals with erythematous raised edges and pale, blanched centres.
- Consider possibility of reflex anoxic seizures.

Management

- **Distinguish acute anaphylaxis from a simple faint**. Feel for a carotid or femoral pulse: if present, of a normal rate and strength, this is probably a faint; if absent or very weak assume this is anaphylactic shock. If in doubt, assume anaphylaxis: fainting is rare in infants.

continued

Treatment of acute anaphylaxis (continued)

- **Place patient in the recovery position**, with the head down. Insert an **oral airway** (size 00 or 0 if 0–1 year, 0 or 1 if 1–5 years, 1 or 2 if 5–12 years and 2, 3 or 4 if an adult).
- **Summon help if readily available**, but not if this will delay treatment for more than a minute or so.
- Administer **adrenaline (1/1,000 i.e. 1 mg/ml)** by deep subcutaneous or intramuscular injection in a dose depending on age:

Less than 6 months	0.05 ml	3–4 years	0.3 ml
6–11 months	0.075 ml	5 years and over	0.5 ml
1 year	0.1 ml	Adult	0.5–1.0 ml
2 years	0.2 ml		

- **Summon help if not already done.**
- If there has been no improvement in 10 minutes, **give a further dose of adrenaline.**
- **Chlorpheniramine (Piriton) should be given subcutaneously in all cases.** The usual preparation is a 1% solution, i.e. 10 mg in 1 ml. The dose is 0.25 mg/kg (0.025 ml/kg) up to a maximum of 20 mg. In an emergency the following is appropriate:

Less than 6 months	1 mg (0.1 ml)	3–7 years	5 mg (0.5 ml)
6–11 months	2 mg (0.2 ml)	Over 7 years	10 mg (1.0 ml)
1–2 years	2.5 mg (0.25 ml)		

- **Another dose of adrenaline** may be repeated after a further 20 minutes.
- **Always admit to hospital** after treatment as there is sometimes a recurrence of symptoms within the first 24 hours.
- **Consult immunization co-ordinator** about further immunizations.

- Children with a **documented history of cerebral damage, a personal history of convulsions or a family history of febrile convulsions or idiopathic epilepsy** are at increased risk of a febrile fit following pertussis and MMR vaccinations. They are not at any greater risk of permanent adverse effects from the vaccines and should receive them. The Department of Health advice is that such children should receive pertussis vaccine. Parents of such children should give them paracetamol for 36–48 hours following vaccination against pertussis. Where a child has an 'evolving neurological disorder' the pertussis vaccine should be temporarily withheld until the picture becomes clear. As the pyrexia following measles/MMR vaccine occurs at an interval of 5–10 days after vaccination, prophylactic paracetamol is not appropriate. The parents should be told what to do in the event of a fever occurring. If such a child is under the care of a paediatrician, and there is any doubt as to whether either vaccine should be given, the paediatrician ought to be consulted first.

Treatment of anaphylaxis

Prevention is better than cure. Check for a history of anaphylaxis or sensitivity to antibiotics. Remember that all available brands of polio vaccine contain penicillin. If in doubt, do not simply advise against immunization; consult the Green Book or call the immunization co-ordinator. You may find it useful to copy the protocol on p. 37–38, and place it where vaccination is carried out. The drugs and equipment mentioned should be easily accessible.

Mythical contraindications

Asthma; eczema; hayfever; snuffles; treatment with antibiotics or locally-acting steroids; being breastfed; mother being pregnant; history of neonatal jaundice; previous clinically diagnosed infection with pertussis, measles, mumps, rubella or polio; failure to thrive; stable neurological conditions such as cerebral palsy and spina bifida; and Down's syndrome have all been cited as reasons for withholding vaccinations. None of these are contraindications to any vaccination.

No allowance should be made for prematurity. The timing of the vaccination programme dates *from birth*, not the expected time of delivery.

Why are high rates of vaccination not achieved more often?

Bearing in mind the very few contraindications that there are to the primary series of vaccinations, uptake rates of the order of 95 per cent are theoretically possible. Why is this level so rarely attained? There are a number of reasons:

- **Low priority**. Acute illnesses and child abuse attract publicity and hence resources at the expense of vaccination programmes.
- **Perceived low risk of diseases**. Many of the diseases against which vaccination is carried out are perceived as being rare. For diphtheria, polio and tetanus this is true, but for others, such as measles and whooping cough, the illnesses are still very common, frequently distressing and sometimes fatal. Table 2.1 shows how commonly these diseases occur in England and Wales. Encephalitis follows measles in between 0.1% and 0.2% of cases and can result in permanent disability. Mumps is the most common cause of aseptic meningitis and is a significant cause of sensorineural hearing loss in children.

Table 2.1. Notifications (and deaths) from vaccine-preventable diseases reported to ONS for the years 1990–5. Deaths are shown in brackets.

Disease	1990	1991	1992	1993	1994	1995
Diphtheria	2(0)	2(0)	8(0)	6(0)	9(2)	12(1)
Hib meningitis	431(26)	417(22)	484(21)	168(6)	52(1)	51(0)
Measles	13,302(1)	9,680(1)	10,268(2)	9,612(4)	16,375(1)	7,768(1)
Mumps	4,277	2,924	2,412	2,153	2,494	1,936
Pertussis	15,286(7)	5,201(0)	2,309(1)	4,091(0)	3,964(3)	1,869(2)
Rubella	11,491(–)	7,174	6,212	9,724	6,326	6,196
Tetanus	9(1)	8(3)	6(1)	8(3)	3(0)	6(2)
Tuberculosis	5,204(390)	5,437(422)	5,799(418)	5,921(423)	5,591(418)	5,608(447)

While polio is rare in this country, it is still very common in developing countries. The disease may be acquired by infants travelling to such countries before they have been immunized.

- **Vaccination not seen as a positive activity**. Undue attention has been given to the very rare adverse effects of vaccination without pointing out the hazards of the diseases. Professionals seem to worry about being blamed for the adverse effects of a vaccination they have given, but are unconcerned by the far commoner situation of a vaccine being withheld for spurious reasons and the child suffering the ill effects of a preventable disease.

Recent evidence suggests that pertussis vaccine rarely, if ever, causes any permanent harmful effects. In fact, recently published data from one of the British birth cohort studies showed that children who had not been immunized against pertussis were *more* likely to be intellectually retarded by the age of 5.

- **Lack of responsibility**. Vaccination is undertaken by GPs and the Community Child Health Services. Until recently, neither had overall responsibility. Thus low uptake rates could be, and often were, blamed on someone else. With the appointment of District immunization co-ordinators this should no longer be the case. The co-ordinator should be willing to offer any practice advice on setting up or improving an immunization programme and to help in individual 'problem' cases where there is doubt as to whether or not a child should be vaccinated.

- **Poor education**. The abundance of mythical contraindications and their propagation by professionals and public alike has caused understandable confusion for some parents. Better training of the professionals and adherence to official guidelines should help to dispel many of these myths. Ready access to a local expert who can offer speedy advice is often found to be helpful. Many Districts provides courses for doctors and nurses.

  Some Districts have Immunization Advice Clinics where children can be referred if there is doubt as to what vaccinations they should be given.

- **Poor information transfer**. Many parents will bring their children for vaccination with little prompting. However, a significant number forget or are reluctant and therefore need reminding. This cannot be done unless accurate records are kept and there is adequate transfer of data between all the professionals involved, i.e. health authorities, GPs, health visitors, etc. Only in this way can individual parents—and their doctors—be reminded of overdue vaccinations.

  Without efficient and speedy feedback, it is impossible to monitor the service being provided and attend to any inadequacies. Feedback to professionals at the grass roots allows them to monitor their own performance in comparison with others and to be alerted to any decline in uptake.

- **Inflexibility**. Vaccinations should be performed not only by the doctor at set times during the day or week, but by any suitably trained person, doctor or nurse, whenever and for whatever reason a child is brought to see that professional, assuming the child is due for vaccination and no real contraindication exists. Practice nurses, clinic nurses and health visitors should all be trained to advise about and give vaccinations, without a doctor being present. If a child is a few days early for a vaccination it should not be put off. On any occasion that a child is seen the vaccination history should be ascertained and any gaps in the programme completed. MMR, DTP and polio vaccines can all be given together, as can Hib and MMR or Hib, DTP and polio.

Opportunistic vaccination is one of the best ways of increasing uptake rates.

Childhood vaccination: a checklist for staff

For all vaccines

- **Is the child acutely unwell with a fever or systemic upset?** If so, postpone the immunization until better.
- **Has the child had a severe reaction (as defined in the 'Green Book') to a previous dose of one of the vaccines about to be given?** If so, discuss with local paediatrician or immunization co-ordinator.

For polio vaccine

- **Is the child or a household member immunosuppressed?** If so, substitute inactivated vaccine (IPV) for the usual oral live vaccine (OPV).
- **Is the child or a household member HIV-positive?** If so, consult local policy about whether IPV should be substituted for OPV.
- **Is the child suffering from acute diarrhoea or vomiting?** If so, postpone vaccination until better.
- **Has the child received immunoglobulin within the last 3 months?** If so, postpone until a full 3 months have elapsed.

For pertussis vaccine

- **Is there a personal, or family, history of convulsions?** If so, remember to give advice about the prevention and treatment of fever.
- **Does the child have a still-evolving neurological condition?** If so, consult the paediatrician looking after the child.

For MMR vaccine

- **Is the child immunosuppressed (excluding due to HIV)?** If so, the vaccine should not be given. It is important that all other family members are immune.
- **Has the child been given another live vaccine (including BCG) within the last 3 weeks?** If so, postpone until a full 3 weeks have elapsed.
- **Has the child ever had an anaphylactic reaction to egg?** If so, discuss with local paediatrician or immunization co-ordinator.
- **Has the child received immunoglobulin within the last 3 months?** If so, postpone until a full 3 months have elapsed.
- **Is the child allergic to kanamycin or neomycin?** If so, discuss with local paediatrician or immunization co-ordinator.

NB Pregnancy should be avoided for 1 month.

continued

Childhood vaccination (continued)

For rubella vaccine

As for MMR except that an anaphylactic reaction to eggs is irrelevant.

For BCG vaccine

- **Is the child 3 months of age or older?** If so, BCG should only be performed after a Heaf or Mantoux test.
- **Is the child HIV positive?** If so, the vaccine should not be given.
- **Is the child immunosuppressed?** If so, the vaccine should not be given.
- **Has the child been given another live vaccine (excluding polio) within the last 3 weeks?** If so, postpone until a full 3 weeks have elapsed.

When non-medical staff take on the responsibility for giving immunizations, they may appreciate the opportunity to attend a short locally organized training course. Where nurses are to give immunizations without a prescription it is essential that they are covered by a 'group protocol'.

Group protocol

A group protocol is a specific written instruction for the supply or administration of named vaccines under specified circumstances. It replaces the need for individual prescriptions. Patient safety must not be compromised and such protocols should not normally include new drugs under intensive monitoring and subject to special adverse re-action reporting requirements (the Black Triangle scheme); unlicensed medicines, e.g. acellular pertussis and IPV in UK; medicines used outside their licensed indications; medicines being used in clinical trials.

Development of the protocol

The protocol should be drawn up by a group including a doctor, pharmacist and at least one representative of each of the professional groups likely to be involved in giving the immunizations covered. This will usually include health visitors, school nurses and practice nurses. It should be approved by the relevant local professional advisory committees and clinical managers.

The content

- The qualifications and training required of staff, e.g. a nurse giving immunizations, should hold a basic qualification and have attended a course on immunization.
- Necessary updating.

continued

Group protocol (continued)

- The criteria for eligibility for vaccination and any exclusions (reference could be made to a checklist such as that on p. 41).
- All the vaccines included in the protocol should be listed. It is not necessary to list doses, route of administration, etc. Cross refer to the Green Book.
- Details of the means by which the administration of the vaccine is to be recorded.
- Action to be taken where a vaccine is refused.
- Identification, management and follow-up of adverse events.
- Arrangements for regular review, monitoring and audit.
- The names of the professionals drawing up the protocol should be stated as should the professional advisory groups and managers giving approval to it.
- The protocol should be dated and signed.

Implementation

- All professionals operating under the protocol should be named and have evidence of competence in the relevant skills and knowledge.
- Participants should be approved by their professional managers.
- Participants must not act beyond their professional competence.
- Participants should sign a copy of the protocol and be provided with written evidence that they are authorized to operate under the protocol.
- A copy of the protocol should be available in the clinical setting in which it operates.
- Arrangements must be in place to modify the protocol in the light of any new data or recommendations.

Source: DoH (1998) *Review of Prescribing, Supply & Administration of Medicines. A Report on the Supply and Administration of Medicines under Group Protocols*. Report of a committee chaired by Dr June Crown, DoH, London.

Commonly asked questions

Q. A child is adopted and the family history is not known—what immunizations should he receive?

A. He should receive all the vaccinations appropriate to his age. The only factor that may be of relevance is the HIV status of the mother. If there is any evidence to suggest that the mother may be HIV-positive, the adoption agency should be consulted.

Q. A child comes from abroad and the immunization status is unknown—what vaccinations should be receive?

A. Assume the child has only received those vaccinations for which there is documentary evidence and give full courses of the remainder.

Q. A course of vaccinations is interrupted by a longer interval than is recommended—should the course be restarted?

A. A course never needs restarting. The remaining dose(s) should be given at the same intervals as would have been appropriate had the course not been interrupted.

Q. Should a child receive one or more polio vaccinations before he is allowed to go swimming?

A. Polio has not been transmitted via swimming pools in the UK. The situation may be different in swimming baths or natural bodies of water in developing countries.

Q. A child has had a disease—should he receive the vaccination against that disease?

A. Only when there is microbiological proof that a child has had a disease should consideration be given to omitting the corresponding vaccine. It is unlikely that a child will have this level of proof of past infection with mumps, measles and rubella, and so MMR should rarely be omitted on these grounds.

   Even if a child has had a microbiologically proven infection he should still be given the vaccine as immunity cannot always be guaranteed after the illness. **No harm will come by vaccinating a child against a disease he has already had.** The only exception to this is BCG which should not be given to someone who has had TB.

Q. Can more than one vaccine be given at the same time?

A. MMR, DTP, polio (IPV or OPV) and hepatitis can be given together, without any increase in adverse effects or reduction in efficacy. The same applies for DTP, polio and Hib, as well as for Hib and MMR. Each injection should be given at a separate site. Some brands of DTP and Hib vaccines can be mixed in the same syringe just before administration and are usually dispensed in the same package. With this exception, no vaccines should be mixed in the same syringe.

Q. A child vomits soon after being given polio drops—should another dose be given?

A. The dose should be repeated if he vomits within 1 hour of the dose.

Q. The 'Statement of Fees and Allowances' (SFA) authorizes payment for tetanus vaccination given every five years, whereas the current Department of Health guidelines 'Immunization against Infectious Disease', recommend that tetanus boosters should only be given every 10 years. Which is correct?

A. There are a number of such anomalies. The SFA details what will attract remuneration, while the guidelines suggest the optimal course of action for the patient. The DoH guidelines should be followed.

Q. The Department of Health guidelines are different from the manufacturer's literature. Which is correct?

A. The manufacturer's literature is based on the original product licence and is often very conservative. The DoH guidelines are more likely to take account of experience since the vaccine was introduced and should be followed in preference to anything else.

Q. A child develops a nodule at the site of a DTP injection. Is this a contra-indication to further doses?

A. Such nodules are quite common and may take months or, less frequently, years to resolve. They are not a contraindication to further doses. They may be more common with injections given too superficially and extra care should be taken with subsequent injections.

Q.   A parent had a 'bad reaction' to a particular vaccine. Should her child receive the vaccine?

A.   There is no convincing evidence that reactions to vaccines run in families and, in any case, it may be difficult to be sure that an event happening at the time of a vaccination is in any way related to the vaccination. A family history is therefore not relevant unless the suspected reaction was a fit, in which case it would be appropriate to recommend that the child should receive an antipyretic after DTP.

Q.   Is recent immunization a contraindication to surgery such as tonsillectomy?

A.   No.

Q.   Is there is a risk of MMR vaccine causing meningitis?

A.   There have been some cases of mild transient meningitis with the Urabe strain of mumps vaccine virus which has now been withdrawn. The MMR vaccines in use in the UK contain the Jeryl Lynn or a closely related strain. The rate of meningitis due to this strain of mumps virus is very low. Note that meningitis occurs in 80% of natural mumps and can be severe; vaccine cases have been mild and have left no sequelae.

Q.   A relative has inflammatory bowel disease. Should the MMR vaccine be withheld?

A.   The hypothesis that measles or MMR vaccines are linked to inflammatory bowel disease have been disproved. This family history is not relevant and the vaccine should be given.

Q.   Should childhood immunizations be made compulsory as in the USA?

A.   In many states it is compulsory for a child to be immunized before school entry. Overall take-up rates are no better than those in Scandinavian countries where immunization is voluntary. More importantly, the take-up rates in 2-year-old children are significantly lower than in the UK. Professional knowledge and enthusiasm are much more effective than compulsion.

Q.   Is there any tissue or protein from cattle in BCG?

A.   No.

Prevention of infectious disease: (b) awareness

Children die or suffer avoidable damage each year because healthcare staff forget that infections can still kill. This section highlights some potentially lethal conditions which are uncommon in the experience of the individual GP, yet need prompt recognition and referral.

Recognizing the sick baby

The 'Baby Check' score was devised to help people decide which babies are ill and which are not. Opinions vary about the value of the scoring system but the criteria used are certainly helpful (available from the Child Growth Foundation, address on p. xiii).

Urinary tract infection

A urinary tract infection in older children usually presents either with frequency and pain, or as an ill child with a high fever, abdominal and/or loin pain. Diagnosis is much more difficult in the first year of life but is also more important because of renal scars and invasive or systemic illness. Consider the diagnosis in any unwell infant, particularly with a temperature over 40 degrees, whether or not you can identify symptoms related to the urinary tract. Unless you can find some other unequivocal source of the infection (beware of slightly red throat or ears) it is important to get a urine culture, preferably before starting antibiotics, and a blood count and blood culture may also be advised. It is very difficult to get an adequate urine specimen in the home or in most health centres, so optimum management of the unwell infant with unexplained high fever usually requires a visit to the hospital emergency department.

Tuberculosis

BCG should be offered to all high risk neonates. The definition of 'high risk' may vary according to local circumstances, but will usually refer to any child in contact with a case and may also include any child whose family comes from an area with an incidence of 40 or more cases per 100,000 population. This includes the Indian sub-continent, China, Africa, Yemen and the Caribbean. Heaf testing, followed by immunization where needed, should be carried out on newly arrived immigrant children from that region.

In young children, tuberculosis may present with TB meningitis, which often causes severe brain damage even if the child survives. There have been many cases of TB meningitis which can be traced to an adult who was not even unwell. TB occurs in persons of all races and ages; it is not confined to people from the Indian sub-continent or the homeless alcoholic. Energetic, urgent contact tracing is the most important means of controlling tuberculosis (more important than BCG) and is mandatory whenever a person is found to have TB. A child with TB is not a significant risk to other people but contact tracing is equally vital to discover the source of the infection. Although this is not really the responsibility of the general practitioner, standards of follow-up vary, so ensure that your patients get optimum management: check that the index case has been notified, that the contact tracer has visited all families exposed to the infected person and that agreed guidelines have been followed.

Meningococcal disease

In 1992, 100 children died from this disease. Mortality can be reduced by improved early treatment. Any child with a short history of a fever and a purpuric rash should be given intramuscular penicillin at once and transferred to hospital as an emergency. The presence or absence of classical signs of meningitis is irrelevant. In some children, there is a transient rash early in the illness which is maculopapular and not purpuric. The risk of anaphylaxis is tiny compared with the dangers of the disease. Crystapen (benzylpenicillin) is stable over several years and should be kept in the emergency bag. The dose is 300 mg (1/2 M unit) for infants under 1 year; 600 mg for children aged 1–10 years.

Prophylaxis for meningitis contacts

This will usually be arranged by the hospital where the patient is admitted, or by the Consultant in Communicable Disease Control; but the GP may be asked to write the prescription and anxious parents will expect him to know what should be done.

Needle stick injuries

Children may find needles on rubbish tips or even in their own gardens. The parents will be concerned that they may have been discarded by drug users and might therefore cause AIDS. The risk of hepatitis B is greater than that of AIDS, but both are unlikely because neither virus is likely to survive for long in this situation. The current advice is to offer an accelerated course of hepatitis B vaccine (*see* Green Book). It is probably sensible to refer such children to the nearest A & E department, where advice can also be offered on testing for HIV and post-exposure prophylaxis with Zidovidine, which probably needs to be given within one hour of exposure to be effective.

Educational visits to farms and zoos

These are a potential source of infectious diseases, especially gastrointestinal infections, and accidents are also a hazard. Simple precautions can increase safety. It is undesirable and unnecessary to prevent children from handling the animals, but they should be under close supervision. Food and drink should not be consumed in close proximity to animals and the children *must* wash their hands first. The Health & Safety Executive has recently produced advice on farm visits for farmers and teachers (AIS23).

Preventing infections in nurseries and primary schools

Skin diseases, infestations, diarrhoeal illnesses, hepatitis A, congenital cytomegalovirus infections and meningitis may worry parents. Many areas have guidelines to minimize the risk of infection. These may be obtained from the community paediatrician or department of public health medicine. At the time of writing the Department for Education and Employment was making available new guidance on infection control in schools and nurseries.

Food hygiene

The incidence of gastroenteritis could be reduced by better food hygiene in the home. The health visitor may be able to provide the appropriate health education.

Kawasaki disease

This exotic sounding infection is not rare. The features are continuing fever, a rash, lymphadenopathy, sore mouth, redness and swelling of the hands and feet, and peeling of the fingers and toes. The child is *extremely* miserable. Early identification

Prophylaxis for contacts of meningococcal and Haemophilus infections

The spectre of meningitis always strikes fear into the hearts of parents. In fact it is unusual for secondary cases to occur, even within families. Remember that it is the septicaemic form of meningococcal disease that has the high mortality rather than meningitis. What follows is advice that is current at the time of writing. **Before treating contacts with antibiotics or vaccine, always consult the local Consultant in Communicable Disease Control (CCDC).**

Meningococcus:

- The highest attack rates are in the age group 1–4 years.
- Antibiotic treatment should be offered to all household contacts and boy/girl friends as soon as possible. This would include boarders in the same dormitory, but not other school or nursery contacts. If the organism is found to be type A, C, W137 or Y, the appropriate vaccine should be given.
- The antibiotic of choice is rifampicin: 10 mg/kg every 12 hours for 2 days (5 mg/kg if < 1 month old) to a maximum 600 mg/dose.* Ciprofloxacin is an unlicensed alternative. Ceftriaxone as a single dose of 250 mg should be used in pregnant women.
- Antibiotic prophylaxis is usually only given to a wider group when two or more cases of the same strain have occurred within the same setting over a short period of time. This should never be done except on the advice of the CCDC, who will often wish to seek national guidance.

Haemophilus:

All unimmunized children under 4 years should be vaccinated as soon as possible.

- Antibiotic prophylaxis is not indicated if all household contacts under 4 years old are fully immunized.
- In households where one or more children are not completely vaccinated, antibiotic prophylaxis should be offered to all home contacts irrespective of age and immunization status.
- The antibiotic of choice is rifampicin: 20 mg/kg once daily for 4 days (10 mg/kg if <1 month old) to a maximum of 600 mg/dose.*
- Antibiotic prophylaxis is usually only given to contacts at play-group, nursery or crèche when two or more cases have occurred within the same setting within 120 days. This should never be done except on the advice of the CCDC, who will often wish to seek national guidance.

* Don't forget to warn women that rifampicin inactivates the oral contraceptive pill for the rest of the cycle.

NB Recommendations change as new evidence appears; check whenever possible with local experts.

Prevention of gastroenteritits

- All mothers should wash their hands with soap:
  - Before breastfeeding.
  - After using the toilet.
  - After changing the nappies of other infants or wiping toddlers' bottoms.
  - After handling raw meat, poultry or eggs.
- Raw meat, *particularly poultry*, often carries bacteria and mothers should:
  - Prepare such foods on a separate surface if possible OR clean the surface, preferably with bleach, before preparing other foods which are not going to be cooked.
  - Store raw foods, *particularly poultry*, at the bottom of the fridge, and keep covered: cooked foods should be at the top.
- Eggs should be well cooked (p. 19).
- Poultry must be well cooked, i.e. not bloody in the middle.
- Unpasteurized milk should NOT be given to babies or young children.
- Toilet handles and taps are a potential source of infection, particularly in day nurseries or large households. They should be wiped with a cloth soaked in diluted bleach.
- Barbecues are a particular hazard—burgers must be well cooked. Beware of using the same tongs for raw and cooked meat.

and referral are vital because of the risk of coronary artery aneurysms. Kawasaki disease is easily mistaken for measles but saliva antibody testing now available at the Public Health Laboratory Service shows that less than 1% of suspected cases in fact have measles. So whenever you think of measles, think of alternatives as well! Consider other viruses, 'slapped cheek syndrome' and drug reactions.

Encephalitis and encephalopathy

The important features are changes in behaviour and consciousness. Sometimes these can be quite subtle and are mistaken for being 'unco-operative' or 'aggressive'. Any child with such complaints should be seen promptly. Deterioration can be rapid and the child should be admitted without hesitation.

Further reading

1. Department of Health (1996) *Immunization Against Infectious Disease*. HMSO, London. This contains the official recommendations which should form the basis of all vaccination practice. An updated edition is sent to all doctors.

2. Jefferson N, Sleight G and MacFarlane A (1987) Immunization of Children by a Nurse Without a Doctor Present. *Br Med J*, **294**, 423–424. A very useful article showing that a suitably trained nurse can carry out immunization without a doctor being on the premises.

3. British Paediatric Association (1996) *Manual of Childhood Infections*. WB Saunders, London. A concise guide to childhood infections. It includes details of diagnosis, management and prevention of infectious diseases in children.

4. Nicoll A and Hull D (1984) Immunization Misinformation. Lancet, **ii**, 1215–1216. Details many of the mythical contraindications to immunization.

5. Nicoll A, Elliman D and Begg NT (1989) Immunization: Causes of Failure and Strategies for Success. *Br Med J*, **299**, 808–812.

6. Bedford H and Elliman D (1998) *Childhood Immunisation: a review for parents and carers*. Health Education Authority, London. A useful detailed guide for parents who want more information on immunization. Also suitable for members of the primary healthcare team.

7. Factsheets, available from the HEA cover polio, MMR and BCG immunizations. Further factsheets covering the other routine immunizations are in preparation.

Information about immunization requirements and anti-malarial precautions for individual countries can be obtained from British Airways Travel (Telephone 0171 831 5333). Prescribing details for vaccines for travel should be obtained from the DoH guide to immunization and for anti-malarial prophylaxis from the British National Formulary.

Leaflets and posters may be obtained from the local Health Promotion Unit or from some of the vaccine manufacturers, e.g. Merieux UK Ltd (01628 785291) and Lederle Praxis (01329 224 000).

Prevention of accidents in childhood

Accident—'an unpremeditated event resulting in recognizable injury' (World Health Organization, 1957).

Accidents are the commonest cause of death in children aged between 1 and 14, accounting for half of all deaths. Two children are killed in accidents every day and 10,000 are permanently disabled each year. Each year one in six children attend hospital accident and emergency departments. Accidents are responsible for 20 per cent of hospital paediatric admissions. This represents an enormous amount of suffering for children and families and costs the NHS nearly £150 million a year.

The fatalities for England and Wales in 1987 can be broken down as follows:

Transport accidents	
vehicle occupants	80
pedestrians	214
pedal cyclists	63
other	24
Total	381
Home accidents	
burns and scalds	89
suffocation	33
drowning	20
falls	11
poisoning	7
other	37
Total	197

Other locations

drowning	27
falls	21
other	62
Total	110
Total all accidents	**688**

The pattern of accidents varies with age, in keeping with the child's development and exposure to new hazards. Prevention can be incorporated into Child Health Surveillance at every stage and while general advice can be given, this will have more impact if it is related specifically to the individual child's environment. For this reason the primary health care team, with its intimate knowledge of the child, his family and the home, is in an ideal position to offer such advice.

The programme of accident prevention may need to be adjusted to fit in with the pattern of surveillance in individual practices. Whenever a home visit is made or a child is seen following an accident, advice should be reinforced. Parents should know how and where to get equipment and to whom they can turn for further advice, e.g. housing department.

After 5 years old, children spend more time out of the supervision of adults. Even if with an adult, the level of supervision is much less and it is therefore very important that they are taught to be responsible in their behaviour.

Children should be taught **road safety**, commensurate with their age and development. Many deaths are caused by children running out into the road when playing. They should only play in allotted areas, where traffic is banned. Many parents underestimate the maturity necessary for children to be safe as pedestrians. When they reach an age to ride a bicycle on the road, they should take a cycling proficiency course first. The use of helmets should be encouraged.

Road accidents are far more common in deprived areas. 'Black spots' are not relevant in childhood pedestrian accidents. The most effective preventive measures are (a) reducing the speed of traffic by road engineering projects and (b) providing safe play areas and activities, particularly after school and in the holidays. All health professionals should support investment in such schemes.

Drowning is a significant cause of death and all children should be taught to swim as soon as possible. As with all accidents, particular care should be taken when children are away from home, where adequate safety precautions may not be in operation. Children of less than secondary school age should never swim without an older person being present.

Farms are a dangerous environment for children, particularly toddlers and teenagers. Common causes of **farm accidents** include tractors and power attachments, falling objects (climbing on unsecured tractor wheels, gates, etc.), falls from buildings (barns, outbuildings), drowning (tanks, troughs), crushing and asphyxia (piles of sacks, silos, manure heaps).

Along with advice about accident prevention, parents should be taught what to do when an accident occurs. Topics that should be covered include first aid treatment of burns and scalds; what to do in suspected poisoning; control of bleeding; and simple resuscitation.

Accident prevention

- Provide practical help in carrying out your suggestions (e.g. where to obtain car-seats, how to have window-locks fitted).
- Make use of national campaigns, local news, videos, magazine articles, etc. to reinforce health education messages. A combination of individual contact, written information, practical help and national campaigns backed by legislation is far more effective than any single approach.
- Check to see whether recommended changes have been carried out.

All school age children should also learn the rudiments of first aid and know what to do in the event of an accident. Ideally this should be the responsibility of the school.

Further reading

1. *Basic Principles of Child Accident Prevention: A Guide to Action* (1989) Child Accident Prevention Trust. An excellent guide for professionals.

2. Asher J (1988) *Keep Your Baby Safe*. Penguin Books. A very useful book for parents, covering children up to 3.

3. *Play it Safe: A Guide to Preventing Children's Accidents*. Health Education Authority. A well-illustrated guide to the prevention and treatment of accidents. Produced for parents, but suitable for professionals.

Leaflets and further information may be obtained from the following:

1. Child Accident Prevention Trust, 28 Portland Place, London W1N 4DE. Tel: 0171-636 2545.

2. Department of Transport, Road Safety Division, 2 Marsham Street, London SW1P 3EB. Tel: 0171-276 3000.

3. Department of Trade and Industry, Consumer Safety Unit, CA Division, 10–18 Victoria Street, London SW1H 0NN. Tel: 0171-215 7877.

4. Royal Society for the Prevention of Accidents, Cannon House, The Priory Queensway, Birmingham B4 6BS. Tel: 0121-200 2461.

5. Health Education Authority, Hamilton House, Mabledon Place, London WC1H 9TX. Tel: 0171-383 3833.

Primary prevention of emotional and behavioural problems

Emotional and behavioural problems of early childhood are not always caused by parents but a good proportion are, either because the child responds in a particular way to aberrant parental handling or because the parents' response to a common variation in the child's developing behaviour has the effect of perpetuating and exaggerating it. It makes sense to advise good child-rearing practice and promote competent parenting.

Most parents *are* competent and fall within the general range of commonsense parenting; they may fret about whether they are doing the right thing for their child but the odds are that they are. It is the parents who fall outside the normal range who are likely to contribute to children's emotional and behaviour problems. Of course, they may be forced beyond the normal range by a difficult child and it is rarely right simply to blame the mother (as is often done). More usually the end-result is the product of an interaction between the child's qualities, the personality and knowledge of each parent and the quality of relationships within the family generally.

Within families, it is attitudes and relationships which influence psychological development rather than child-rearing practices alone. Often it is difficult to disentangle the two, but in the majority of families the emphasis should be on quality of family relationships. Whether or not to smack children is therefore a less important question than whether the child can earn praise and affection.

Take the opportunity during surgery and home visits to observe and enquire in order to form an impression as to whether the parents are competent.

Competent parents

- Protect their children from physical harm.
- Attend to their needs for shelter, food, affection, approval, information and advice.
- Keep adult business (sex, marital conflicts, major worries about money etc.) separate from their children.
- Use authority so that they are in charge of their children rather than *vice versa*.
- Respect children's immature status and have a reasonable idea of what this is for each child.
- Set limits of acceptability on their children's behaviour.
- Use a *moderate* number of rules whose purpose can be explained to, and understood by, children.
- Are consistent from one occasion to another, between each other, and between children according to their developmental status.
- Allow their child a measure of autonomy, tailored to developmental status, allowing him to experiment and learn from experience.
- Use praise focused on the child's achievements.
- Justify prohibitions (briefly) and use mainly non-physical punishments.
- Avoid:
  - Threats that cannot be implemented.
  - Using fear as the only disciplinary weapon.
  - Protracted nagging or moaning.
  - Denigrating children.
  - Cruel punishments.
  - Excessive physical punishments.
  - Burdening children with worries which they are not mature enough to cope with.

These statements are derived from systematic studies, not a particular ideological approach. It is not advocacy for a liberal, open approach. Parents who are firm, kind and reasonable have children who are better adjusted than those who allow all emotions to be expressed to anyone, who have no rules, believe in arguing everything through, and who set no limits on children's choices and behaviours.

CHAPTER 3

Secondary prevention

Contents

The value of early detection
   Early detection is important
Early detection of developmental problems
   A systematic approach
   Developmental screening tests
   Primary care decisions
Early detection of hearing loss
   What are you looking for?
   Audiology service
   Detection
   Terms used in hearing assessment
   Clinical evaluation
   Deaf children
Early detection of vision defects
   Early diagnosis
   Definitions
   Terms used in vision assessment
   Refractive errors
   Recent advances in the assessment of vision
   Referral of suspected vision problems
   Children with impaired vision
Early detection of emotional and behavioural disorders: the child
Early detection of emotional and behavioural disorders: the family
   Issues in normal family functioning
   Risk factors for the development of disturbance
Child mental health surveillance
   A framework for assessment
Making sense of emotional and behavioural problems
Child protection
   Physical abuse
   Sexual abuse
   Emotional abuse and failure to thrive
   Management of a case of suspected child abuse
   The Children Act, 1989
   Children looked after

This section emphasizes the importance of early detection and explains some of the ways by which it may be achieved. Early detection of defects is only one of the goals of child health promotion programmes and is not necessarily the most important. However, parents prefer to know about their child's problems as soon as possible; they want health professionals to take their concerns seriously; they expect routine checks and tests to be done competently; they need sensible advice and appropriate intervention.

The value of early detection

Early detection is important

- Early treatment may reduce or even avoid permanent damage in some conditions.
- An early diagnosis may allow genetic counselling thus avoiding the birth of another handicapped child.
- The most important reason is that **parents value early diagnosis**. This is probably because it is easier to come to terms with a serious problem in a young baby than in an older child who has already acquired a personality and a shared life with the parents. **It is not a kindness to keep parents in ignorance and leave them to find out for themselves that their child is abnormal.**

Repeated detailed examination and developmental testing of all children (developmental screening) is not necessarily the best way of achieving early diagnosis.

Early diagnosis is achieved by:

- Careful examination of all neonates and a repeat examination at 6–8 weeks of age.
- Specialist follow-up of high risk babies and children (e.g. those thought to have suffered brain injury due to periventricular haemorrhage or meningitis).
- **Responding promptly to parents' worries is the most economic and effective single method of early detection.** Parents often realize something is wrong with the child's development or health even though they cannot work out exactly what it is.

In today's small nuclear families, parents do not necessarily begin their family life with much experience of small children, nor do they always have such easy access to the wisdom of grandparents as their own parents would have done. Nevertheless, most learn quickly. They watch their children playing at nursery and playgroup and discuss them with the staff; they talk to friends and neighbours; listen to grandparents; watch television programmes and read magazines. (The media have done much to raise public knowledge about handicap in childhood.) By the time they bring a child to the doctor or health visitor with a concern about health, growth or development they have thought about the suspected problem very carefully.

It follows that if parents say something is wrong, you should assume that they are correct until proved otherwise. Never assume that parents are fussy, overanxious or neurotic.

A child health programme should facilitate the discovery of abnormality by providing advice and easy access to expert opinion. Where parents are uncertain or do not find it easy to face the possibility of some serious problem, the support of a professional is often invaluable. Since there is rarely great urgency about the diagnosis of a chronic problem, a few discussions spread over several weeks often enable them to accept and make use of specialist referral.

The term **screening** refers to the examination of apparently healthy children to distinguish those who probably have a condition from those who probably do not. The aim of a screening programme is to examine *all* the children at risk. This usually means the entire population of children of a particular age, but in some cases selected high-risk groups only may be offered the test. The role of screening tests in child health is to detect conditions that might otherwise be overlooked by both parent and professional unless a specific search is undertaken.

Opportunistic screening means making use of contacts between child and professional to evaluate the child's health and development. In contrast to population screening, with opportunistic screening the contact is initiated by the parents because of some concern or anxiety.

Early detection of developmental problems

A systematic approach

It is convenient to review development under the following headings:

- Gross motor; sitting, standing, walking, running.
- Fine motor; handling toys, stacking bricks, doing buttons.
- Speech and language, including hearing.
- Social behaviour.

Note that a difficulty or delay in any aspect of development must be regarded as a **symptom requiring a differential diagnosis**. For example, poor motor co-ordination might be due to visual impairment or general backwardness, as well as conditions that specifically affect movement such as cerebral palsy. Poor co-ordination is *not* a diagnosis.

Ask the parents!

The best way to find out about a child's development is to ask the parents. Questions must be precise and parents must not be allowed to get away with vague answers!

Parents are usually surprisingly objective in their observations and rarely exaggerate, but they do *not* always understand the significance of what they see. For instance, they may describe the inability of a three-year-old to understand simple instructions, but *not* realize that this is probably abnormal. When parents do not seem able to make accurate observations, it may be useful to ask them what the playgroup leader or nursery nurse thinks. People who spend their days working with a wide variety of children are usually very astute in recognizing abnormalities.

Parents are much better at telling you about **current** abilities than about past milestones. Do not waste a lot of time trying to establish exactly when a child first sat or walked.

Check that the parents' description of what the child does is supported by observation. Watch the child in the playroom, waiting room or whenever the opportunity arises. Use what you see as a talking point with the parents.

Developmental screening tests

Simple screening tests such as the Denver Developmental Screening Test (*see* Figure 3.1) are widely used. But we do not recommend them for **routine** use because:

- The range of normality is so wide that many of the children whose development falls outside the accepted 'norms' are nevertheless normal. The concept of 'pass' or 'fail' intrinsic to a screening test is restrictive and constrains professional judgement.
- Conversely, some children with significant handicapping conditions develop apparently 'normally' as assessed by tests, at least within the first year or two.
- Parents' perceptions of normal development vary widely according to their expectations of their children and of life in general. Thus parents in poor circumstances may regard their child's poor speech as the least of their problems, whereas prosperous middle-class parents will go to great lengths to deal with even trivial difficulties. Screening tests cannot take account of this variation.
- It is more profitable to help parents to:
  - Anticipate developmental difficulties.
  - Take action to improve the child's environment.
  - Increase their own ability to recognize and respond to any problems that occur.
- In reality, the factor which has the most effect on referral of children with suspected developmental problems is probably the availability of resources to deal with them.

Provided that these limitations are recognized, there is no reason why staff who are not yet familiar with child development should not use a developmental chart or test as a way of increasing their knowledge and competence. The Denver Test, which is reproduced in Figure 3.1, provides a convenient summary of developmental progress and includes useful information about the *range* of ages at which abilities are usually acquired. The *Schedule of Growing Skills* (publisher NFER-Nelson) is also useful.

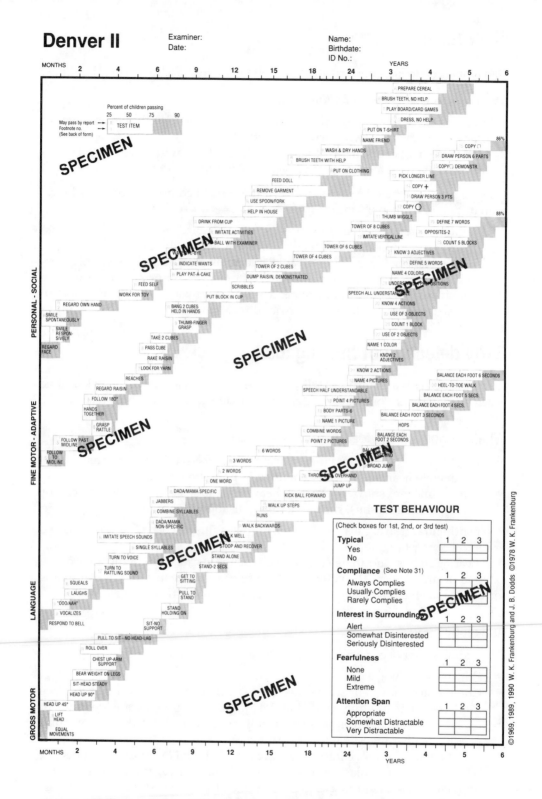

Available from the Test Agency, Cournswood House, Clappins Lane, North Dean, High Wycombe, HP14 4NW (Telephone 01494 563384).

Figure 3.1. Denver Developmental Screening Test.

Primary care decisions

The aim is to make two clinical decisions.

1. Is there likely to be a significant abnormality in this child's development or behaviour; and if so, what aspects are affected?
2. Are there any factors in this child's development or environment which might constructively be altered or improved?

If the answer to either question is YES, a more detailed assessment may be required. You must then decide:

3. Should you refer the child onwards for more detailed assessment and if so, to whom? Or should you manage the problem within the primary care team? This depends on the level of skill available in the practice and on ease of access to specialist services. Many health visitors are competent to deal with common management problems and many more can acquire the necessary skills if appropriate training is provided.

Early detection of hearing loss

A hearing defect is a hidden disability and even a very deaf baby may look as if he is behaving normally, because of the ability to understand situations by using clues.

What are you looking for?

*   Sensorineural hearing loss (nerve deafness). Affects 1–2:1000 children.
*   Conductive hearing loss; very common in pre-school children.
*   Some children show abnormal hearing responses for neurological or developmental reasons, such as learning disability* or autism.

A **sensorineural** hearing loss is caused by a defect in the cochlea, auditory nerve or central connections.

A hearing loss is said to be **conductive** when it is caused by a disorder of the external or middle ear. The commonest cause of a conductive loss in children is secretory otitis media (SOM), also known as otitis with effusion or glue ear.

Audiology service

The audiology service is usually organized in three tiers:

*   Primary screening.
*   Community referral or second tier clinics: the precise role varies from place to place—some are fully staffed and equipped and provide a wide range of expert services, whereas others act only as a filter and refer on any child needing further investigation or treatment.
*   Consultant (third tier) clinics: these are usually based in a hospital. At district level they provide diagnostic services and support early intervention programmes. Cases requiring complex genetic or ENT investigations or assessment for cochlear implantation are referred to specialized regional or supra-regional centres.

*Previously called mental handicap.

Detection

No single test can be relied on to find all cases of hearing loss in children. The following strategy is suggested:

- **Neonatal screening** (p. 138).
- At the **8-week examination** the parent is asked about any concerns related to hearing and also any high risk factors for hearing loss. No attempt is made to test the infant's hearing, as no behavioural test is reliable at this age. If the parent is seriously concerned the baby should be referred.
- At any time when the parent is worried there should be easy access to expert testing. In some clinics, self-referral is accepted and delay is therefore kept to a minimum. **When parents suspect a hearing loss, there is a high probability that they are correct.** Unfortunately, parents' conviction that their child has **normal** hearing is not so reliable, though their observations can probably be made more accurate by providing written information about normal hearing behaviour in the Parent Held Record (p. 110).
- Babies who were not screened in the neonatal period should have a **hearing assessment at 6–8 months**. Current policy in most Districts is that this should incorporate the **distraction test** (p. 170), but suitable quiet conditions are essential and a high standard of testing must be set and maintained by constant vigilance and monitoring. If this is not possible the test should not be done. In some Districts the distraction test has been discontinued and more reliance is placed on parental education and awareness, together with observation of the baby's hearing responses to voice and environmental sounds and his communicative behaviour.
- Surveillance of children between 2 and 5 years should focus on the discovery of **problems in language acquisition and on behavioural disorder**. If there is doubt about the hearing, delay in language development, or the presence of **persistent middle ear problems**, a speech discrimination test may be done by primary care staff if adequately trained, otherwise the child should be referred to the second tier clinic.
- All **school entrants** should have an audiometric test (the 'sweep' test), and/or a speech discrimination test, and/or an impedance test, according to local policy.
- Children found to have **serious developmental problems** such as cerebral palsy, mental handicap or vision defect should routinely be referred for full hearing assessment.
- Children at **high risk of persistent 'glue ear'** should be checked regularly, i.e. those with Down's, Turner's and Williams' syndromes, cleft palate (even after repair), Pierre Robin syndrome and other craniofacial malformations.
- Children under the age of 5 who have had **acute bacterial meningitis or meningococcal septicaemia** should have a hearing test *soon* after recovery, and some authorities also suggest that children who have had **measles** and **mumps** should be tested.

The above strategy can only work if it is possible for primary care staff to refer promptly to a consultant or to a community audiology service. A **full audiological service** is imperative for those children found to have a sensorineural hearing loss. This should include medical and educational rehabilitation with the provision of teaching and appropriate amplification; input from a specialist speech and language therapist; paediatric examination; support services; advice about financial help and voluntary organizations; genetic counselling.

Terms used in hearing assessment

The **intensity** of a sound is measured in decibels (dB). **Loudness** is the subjective impression of intensity. 0 dB is the hearing threshold of the average person (*not* the absence of sound), 50–60 dB is the intensity of a conversational voice; 100–105 dB might be the intensity of a shout; and 140 dB is the threshold of pain. Intensity is measured using a **sound-level meter**.

A person with impaired hearing only hears sound when it is raised above the normal threshold of 0 dB. The sound intensity needed to exceed the threshold is the **hearing loss** for that ear. For example, a person who hears no sound quieter than 80 dB has a hearing loss of 80 dB. Hearing loss is measured with an **audiometer**.

Frequency is measured in cycles per second or Hertz (Hz). **Pitch** is the subjective impression of frequency. The human ear can detect sounds of between 16 Hz and 20,000 Hz, but in clinical practice tests are confined to the speech frequencies, usually 250–8000 Hz.

Vowel sounds tend to be low frequency sounds (250–1000 Hz) and **consonants** are usually high frequency; the ones with the highest frequency are ss, sh, f and v.

A **whisper** has a frequency range above 1000 Hz whereas a **voice**, however quiet, contains low frequency components of 250–1000 Hz.

Clinical evaluation

This consists of:

- The history—risk factors for hearing loss, parents' observations.
- Observation of behaviour.
- Behavioural testing—i.e. tests of hearing that rely on some form of response from the child.
- Physical examination. **The clinical evaluation of hearing at different ages is described in detail on pp. 169 and 216.**

Objective tests

These are methods of assessing hearing without the co-operation of the subject, and are particularly valuable for testing very young or handicapped children. They include brainstem evoked response audiometry (BSER), and the method of otoacoustic emissions ('cochlear echo'). Both techniques require expensive equipment and considerable skill in their performance and interpretation. Sedation is not needed in infants but may be needed in older children. Simplified versions of the techniques are available for screening. This is mainly used for high risk populations but universal neonatal screening is now feasible (see p. 138).

Impedance measurement (tympanometry) is a technique of estimating the mechanical properties of the middle ear. The stiffness or impedance of the eardrum and middle ear structures is altered by the presence of fluid or negative pressure in the middle ear cavity. It is therefore a very sensitive way of detecting the presence of SOM.

Impedance measurement does not provide a direct means of detecting hearing loss; its main value is in investigating the site (middle ear versus cochlea or nerve) of a hearing loss already demonstrated by the tests described previously. It is an invaluable tool in the audiology clinic but we do not think it has any place in primary care clinics. Some authorities believe that impedance tests should be introduced as part of the school entrant hearing assessment, but there is as yet no consensus on this point. SOM is so common that it often co-exists with more serious sensorineural deafness and it can be very difficult to recognize such cases.

Deaf children

The diagnosis and follow-up of a child with a sensorineural hearing loss is the responsibility of the audiology clinic. The parents should expect to receive the following:

- An accurate estimate of the severity of the hearing loss as soon as the child's maturity allows this.
- An explanation of the nature of the defect and the reasons why it cannot be cured surgically.
- An honest account of what can and cannot be achieved by hearing aids and by new technology such as cochlear implants.
- A paediatric assessment to exclude any other defects.
- A vision check. Clearly it is more than usually important for the deaf child to have good eyesight.
- Where appropriate, other specialist services, e.g. a regional audiology clinic, genetic clinic etc.
- An introduction to the peripatetic teacher specializing in hearing loss.
- An explanation of the relative merits of oral and signed methods of communication, without any undue bias (there are still some teachers who will not teach signing even to a profoundly deaf child, often with disastrous effects—the child grows up without any effective means of communication and may become psychiatrically disturbed).
- Introduction to social services and voluntary organizations such as the National Deaf Children's Society.

Early detection of vision defects

Serious defects of vision are uncommon. The incidence is around 4 children per 10,000, although this figure does not include all the children with cortical vision defects (*see* below) and is therefore an underestimate. The general practitioner may see only one new case of a congenital handicapping vision defect in his professional lifetime, and even a consultant ophthalmologist at a District General Hospital may see only one or two cases per year. Minor vision problems, on the other hand, are very common; between 5 and 10 per cent of children have a squint, a refractive error, or both.

Early diagnosis

The early diagnosis of eye defects in children is important for several reasons.

- Some conditions need early investigation and treatment, for example retinoblastoma, cataract and glaucoma.
- Eye defects are often accompanied by abnormalities in other organs and therefore early paediatric assessment is advisable.
- Many eye diseases are genetic in origin and early counselling should be offered to avoid the birth of a second handicapped child.
- Severe visual defects affect all areas of development and may also result in secondary behavioural and emotional disturbances, which can be prevented by appropriate management.
- The early diagnosis of squint is important because:
  - It may be a sign of serious ocular or neurological disease.
  - It predisposes to the development of amblyopia.
- The early diagnosis of refractive error is worthwhile because:
  - Impaired visual acuity may affect other aspects of development.
  - It may also predispose to the development of amblyopia.

Definitions

A **serious or disabling defect** can be defined as one which affects the child's vision to the extent that he has difficulty in coping with normal schooling without some form of additional assistance. It corresponds very roughly to a corrected vision of 6/18 or worse (i.e. the best vision obtainable when wearing correct glasses). Other factors also determine the extent to which a particular defect causes a disability; for instance, field defects, photophobia, intelligence and so on. **Partial sight** means that there is some residual vision which can be used for education or work; **blind** means that the person can only use methods for education or work which do not require the use of any vision.

An **ocular defect** is one in which the poor vision is caused by some defect of the eye itself or of the optic nerve.

A **cortical defect** is one in which the abnormality lies in the brain rather than in the eye. It is unusual for the occipital cortex to be damaged in isolation, and more commonly cortical vision defects are associated with other serious neurological problems such as cerebral palsy or mental handicap.

Defects which are seldom disabling though not necessarily trivial include squint, refractive error, amblyopia and ptosis (*see* box).

The Snellen letter charts are the recognized method of ascertaining and recording visual acuity. The standard test is done at a distance of 6 metres between subject and chart. The result is given as a pseudofraction. Thus 6/6 means that the person can read at 6 metres the same as the average person; 6/12 means that the subject can read only at 6 metres the letters which the average person can read at 12 metres.

The term **refractive error** (*see* box) means that the eye is not functioning as a perfect optical system. In other words, the refracting structures of the eye, the lens and cornea, do not bring rays of light to a perfect focus on the retina. It is measured in terms of the correcting lens which must be placed in front of the eye in order to produce a sharp image on the retina.

Terms used in vision assessment

- **Squint** means that the visual axis of one eye is not directed to the same point as the visual axis of the other eye.

- A **pseudosquint** is the illusory appearance of a squint created by broad epicanthic folds. Pseudosquint and true squint can co-exist.

- A **manifest squint** is one which is constantly present.

- A **latent squint** is only evident under conditions of stress such as fatigue, illness or provocative testing.
  Manifest squints are cosmetically unattractive and predispose to the development of amblyopia (p. 225) but latent squints are generally of less significance.

- An **alternating squint** is one in which the child fixates with either eye alternately. It is less likely to lead to amblyopia.

- Some books on child care still state that a squint can be normal up to the age of 6 months. This is misleading; some babies may have a transient loss of conjugate gaze when tracking a close moving object, but a **permanent squint in one eye is never normal**.

- **Ptosis** is drooping of the upper eyelid. It may be unilateral or bilateral. If it is severe enough to occlude the pupil it may cause amblyopia, otherwise its main significance is cosmetic and an occasional association with other paediatric disorders.

- Vision is described in terms of **visual acuity**, which is a measure of the subject's ability to discriminate visual stimuli. The measurement of visual acuity normally requires some form of co-operation or behavioural response from the subject.

Most eyes have a slight degree of long- or short-sightedness, which can be measured by the ophthalmologist with a retinoscope, but there is no exact relationship between this measurement and the visual acuity. The decision as to whether a person has a *significant* degree of refractive error depends on the visual acuity measurement. It is important to remember that when the subject is too young or handicapped to co-operate, the ophthalmologist can determine whether spectacles would produce a sharper image falling on the retina but may have as much difficulty as the non-specialist in measuring visual acuity.

Amblyopia is a condition in which vision is impaired even when any refractive error has been corrected, in spite of there being no disease of the eye or visual pathways.

It can be caused by any condition which prevents a clear image from reaching the retina, for instance, refractive error, particularly when there is a difference between the two eyes (anisometropia), squint or severe ptosis. It occurs only during the period of brain maturation and is therefore only likely to develop in the first seven or eight years of life.

Refractive errors

- In **myopia** or short-sightedness, the subject has difficulty in seeing objects at a distance. Myopia is very uncommon in preschool children but the incidence rises steadily throughout the school years. Severe myopia is a disability both in sport and in classroom work, but there is little evidence that minor degrees of myopia cause any significant inconvenience.

- In **hypermetropia** or long-sightedness, distant objects are perceived clearly but the subject has difficulty in seeing close objects. Children respond to this by increasing accommodation (i.e. the ability to converge the eyes and change the shape of the lens), but sometimes this results in a squint. A deficiency in near visual acuity is therefore unlikely to be the presenting feature of hypermetropia in young people. It is usually discovered when the child presents with a squint (with or without amblyopia).

- **Astigmatism** means that there is a different degree of refraction in the horizontal and vertical axes of the eye and this results in a distorted image.

- **Anisometropia** is the condition in which there is a significant difference in the refractions of the two eyes.

Amblyopia impairs the development of three-dimensional vision, which may cause a minor degree of disability in some sports. If it is severe, the person has effectively only one eye, and will be barred from some careers, such as the Armed Forces, and becomes seriously disabled if so unfortunate as to lose the other eye through disease or accident. A person who has good 3-D vision can be presumed to have no amblyopia and is unlikely to have a significant squint or refractive error. For this reason, tests for 3-D vision have been examined as a means of screening young children for vision defects.

Recent advances in the assessment of vision

Research on the physiology and psychology of visual development has produced a number of promising approaches to the assessment of vision in the very young child. Techniques which have been investigated include refraction of all infants as a screening procedure; the method of forced choice preferential looking, which relies on the infant's preference for novel visual stimuli; various automated methods of refraction.

More research is needed before any of these methods can be considered as a routine screening procedure. Even if the test itself is suitable for widespread use, it remains to be shown that the early detection of vision defects results in an improved outcome, though preliminary results do suggest that the very early diagnosis of refractive error followed by suitable spectacle correction may reduce the incidence of squint and amblyopia.

Referral of suspected vision problems

Children who are too young to co-operate with the standard visual acuity tests should be referred to a community orthoptist or to a children's eye clinic.

Referral to an optometrist is an acceptable alternative for children old enough to perform Snellen visual acuity tests, if the problem appears to be solely one of reduced visual acuity found on routine testing.

If a serious vision defect is suspected at any age, an immediate referral to a consultant ophthalmologist is essential and every effort should be made to obtain an urgent appointment. In practice, a telephone call to a paediatrician may be the fastest route to obtaining this, and also ensures that the child has a complete physical examination. This is important not only because urgent treatment may be needed, but also because the parents will undoubtedly be extremely anxious. Furthermore, lack of normal visual behaviour can also be the presenting feature of more generalized developmental delay or mental handicap syndromes.

Children with impaired vision

Severe visual impairment reduces the rate of early development and may also result in some undesirable secondary phenomena. Social smiling, reaching, hand regard, grasping objects, localization of sound, sitting, the development of object permanence and stranger awareness, the urge to crawl and walk in pursuit of interesting objects are all dependent on vision in the normal infant and are slow to emerge where there is visual handicap. Language development is also delayed in many cases, because the baby is at a disadvantage in learning the association between the objects he perceives and their names. The older child may show excessive echolalia and a tendency to inconsequential chatter as a means of maintaining social contact.

Blind babies sometimes adopt an unusual posture, with the hands inert and resting beside the shoulders. Parents may feel that the child is somewhat slow and unresponsive, indeed they may feel rejected and therefore find it difficult to give the attention that is needed. Lacking the social contact and attention that he needs to make sense of the world around him, the infant may withdraw into self-stimulating procedures such as rocking, head banging or eye poking. Good early counselling and management help to reduce or avoid these various secondary handicapping problems.

It is not surprising, therefore, that the results of developmental examinations are particularly difficult to evaluate in a blind or partially sighted infant. Some degree of developmental delay is expected but one may have to decide whether there are motor or intellectual deficits associated with the vision disorder. This difficulty is commonly encountered because there are many eye conditions which are part of a more generalized developmental disorder. It is advisable to refer to a developmental scale or test which has been developed specifically for the visually handicapped population, for example the Reynell Zinkin Scale.

Primary care staff would not normally expect to be involved in the developmental examination of a child with poor vision, but the following points may be helpful to those who have a **visually handicapped child in their practice**:

- Very few people see enough children with severe visual handicap to acquire much expertise in developmental assessment. The parents may wish to consult with someone who has such experience. This expertise may be available at a Regional Child Development Centre.

- The child's parents and the specialist visiting teacher have a great deal of knowledge about the child's abilities although they may find it difficult to interpret their observations.
- The child is likely to perform considerably better in familiar surroundings and with his own toys and possessions. Lighting and colour contrast may affect the ability to make use of residual vision.
- It is essential to try and establish the approximate level of functional vision before using any play or test materials to investigate intellectual ability.
- Since vision disorders are very often part of a more generalized developmental disorder, it is essential that every child has a full physical examination to look for dysmorphic features and neurological abnormalities.
- Paediatric ophthalmology is a highly specialized field, and a second opinion regarding the diagnosis may be worthwhile.
- The clinical geneticist may have particular skill in recognizing unusual syndromes which may be important from the genetic point of view.
- Assessment of hearing in the visually handicapped infant is particularly difficult because the turning and localizing responses which are normally relied upon are impaired or absent. The child may respond to a sound only by smiling or by cessation of bodily activity. In some cases, electrical response audiometry is the only solution.

Early detection of emotional and behavioural disorders: the child

It is not necessary to get into an argument with yourself as to whether a young child has or has not got an emotional or behavioural disorder, is psychiatrically disordered or psychologically disturbed. All such terms overlap and none of them is absolute. If a child is doing something that is outside the range you would expect for his or her age and circumstances and is either causing or experiencing distress then there is a problem which merits attention. If what they are doing is getting in the way of living a reasonable life, there is similarly a problem. It is better to think in terms of problems, impaired functioning and suffering rather than enter a sterile debate as to whether or not a disorder is present.

Psychological problems may be short-lived and understandable or chronic and perplexing. In many instances, working through the chart in Figure 3.2 will help.

Some elements in the young child represent risk factors for the development of emotional or behavioural problems:

- Difficult temperament (p. 117) or poor fit between the child's temperament and the parents' expectations.
- Low intelligence (high intelligence is a protective factor).
- Delay in speech or language development.
- Brain damage or epilepsy.
- Being a boy.

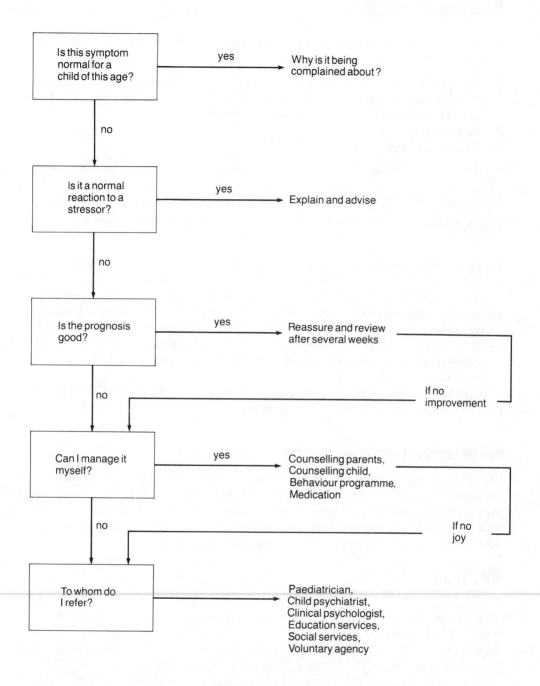

Figure 3.2. Chart to help with working through psychological problems.

Some problems deserve early, active intervention and have a poor prognosis if treated expectantly:

- Any problem that is connected with a poor or abnormal relationship; patterns of relationships are remarkably stable and this will therefore apply to any emotion or behaviour which derives from them.
- Aggression.
- Pervasive hyperactivity.

Early detection of emotional and behavioural disorders: the family

Parents and families may, by various vicissitudes, cause children's psychological problems but not nearly as often as they think they do. Not all children's problems are the result of aberrant parenting and parents, usually, have less influence on children's personality development than they are commonly thought to have. Nevertheless, poor parenting, poor relationships between the child and other family members, unhelpful parental attitudes and practices, and deviant family functioning are the commonest causes of behavioural and emotional disorders in early childhood.

In order to make sense of parenting and family functioning and to identify problems early, some basic concepts are essential.

Issues in normal family functioning

There are, perhaps, two concepts to grasp which relate to normal as well as abnormal families. First the idea of **identification** by which a child takes on himself the attributes of another person, particularly a parent. Secondly the use of ideas derived from **systems theory** (i.e. boundaries and systems) which are used to describe the structure of the family as a functioning unit.

Identification

Early attachment behaviour (clinging and following) subsides during early development with the formation of interpersonal affectional bonds. These are emotions which form the foundations of close, loving relationships. They are characterized by a sense of affection, loyalty and an emotional security in the knowledge of being loved and cherished by the person with whom the bond is formed. These feelings survive geographical separation and therefore make separations possible so that clinging can be abandoned, but a permanent loss of contact with the loved person produces grief. The first relationships a child develops should be characterized by these feelings because they are immensely important in laying the foundations of future relationships, in enabling a secure sense of self to develop, and in learning how to manage anxiety and unhappiness.

Associated with these positive feelings is a strong tendency to take upon oneself the characteristics of the loved person; an identification with them. This aids socialization and development of an adequate sense of self.

Not all identification depends upon attachment formation. It is a common observation that children, or indeed adults, are prone to adopt the characteristics of those who have power over them. Thus a child can identify with a parent who is aggressive to them, becoming aggressive in turn.

Boundaries and systems

One way of thinking about family functioning is to think about a family in terms of different patterns of role and relationship (**systems**). Thus there is always a parenting system (or **subsystem** if one thinks of the whole pattern of roles in the family as one system) which involves the parents in caring for and bringing up their children. In a two-parent family there will be a marital system, and a sibling system when there are several children. Each system has business within it that is not part of other systems. Sex, for example, belongs within the marital system and should not leak out into the parenting system or incest could result.

Around each system and each person in the system is a **boundary** which is impermeable to a greater or lesser degree. Diffuse and inconsistent boundaries can cause problems as can inappropriate ones, as when one parent refuses to let the other parent become involved in looking after a child.

Risk factors for the development of disturbance

Maternal depression

This is a common problem in families of disturbed children, particularly pre-schoolers. Small children of a depressed mother may be uncontained and noisy. Older ones are more likely to be 'parentified' (*see* below). The mother herself may be irritable or inert or both and is likely to be self-preoccupied and inconsistent in her management of the children. Antidepressants may help, but often do not. As a rule, counselling, involving her partner or another relative in active support, building social links outside home and generally taking a social approach to the problem is more likely to succeed. Badly behaved children can exacerbate and perpetuate depression arising for other reasons, so it may be sensible to see if she can be spared the burden of care in some way by arranging playgroups etc. The involvement of a health visitor or social worker can thus be crucial.

Parentification

The child takes on the attributes of a parental role and comforts, reassures and looks after a sick, lonely or depressed parent, being solicitous and helpful to a remarkable degree. Obviously this can be appropriate when a parent is temporarily ill but if the problem is long-standing it is likely to distort personal development as adult anxieties and responsibilities overwhelm the immature child. It can be seen, for example, in many cases of maternal depression, incest and parental alcohol or drug abuse. Only a parent can relieve the child from such a role and many parentified children will not give up readily. Its abandonment by the child is often followed by temporary regression and deterioration in the child's behaviour. It is important to stress to parents that they should be in charge of children and not *vice versa*.

Overprotection

Although this is perhaps the most common criticism of parenting voiced by doctors, it is less common than many imagine. The over-protective parent infantilizes their child. As a result, the child has a narrower range of experiences and fewer opportunities to experiment and solve social problems and feared situations by learning to master them. In consequence, he is likely to be less mature socially and more fearful. It may be coupled with parental indulgence with the consequence that the child becomes a spoilt brat who tyrannizes the home by demanding behaviour, stubbornness and tantrums. The origins of parental overprotection are various:

- Precious child (parental subfertility results in the birth of a very long-awaited baby; a life-threatening illness in infancy has bred the notion of a fragile child).
- Affection is displaced to the child away from the husband because of marital estrangement.
- A mother who was deprived of affection in her own childhood is now compensating for this either by consciously deciding that the same deprivation of love and caring will not happen to her child, or by vicarious identification with the child whom she lavishes care upon, enjoying this at second hand.
- The child is actually resented by the parent who then over-compensates to assuage the guilt.
- The youngest child is usually the last to leave home and will thus leave the parents on their own with each other. They may not look forward to this and unconsciously hang on to him, keeping him a dependent child so that it will be difficult for him to leave.

It is usually wise to see both parents (possibly grandparents too) and explain how overprotection delays social maturation. As in many instances of advising parents, it is better to suggest what they *can do* (such as encouraging the child to make trips away from home to stay with friends) rather than repeatedly emphasize what they should *not* be doing.

Enmeshment

This is a family therapy term which refers to families with an over-close relationship with few boundaries, every member being over-involved with each other's business. In such families, members get upset or anxious on each other's behalf and there are often difficulties over whose feelings belong to whom. Understandably, it is difficult for members to feel themselves to be individuals.

Vicarious satisfaction

Parents may live through their children for the sake of excitement or achievement. Their own disappointments and shortcomings can thus be resolved at second hand. This self-evidently puts a burden on any child who may be encouraged overtly or covertly to do things he would not otherwise do. A more complicated variant is when a parent punishes a child for something which reflects an attribute or activity of their own which they are ashamed of and would like to punish in themselves. Such mechanisms are instances of the mental mechanism of **projection**.

Rejection

The child is disliked, even hated, and in serious cases the parents demand his removal from the family. As a consequence he may react in various ways:

- Stealing from home.
- Adopting a frantically ingratiating stance, writing letters to his parents with declarations of love, buying or stealing lavish presents for them.
- Aggressive, limit-testing behaviour.

It is often associated with evidence of low self-esteem on the part of both parents and child. This seems to breed rigidity on both sides. Rejection is notoriously difficult to reverse but counselling the rejecting parent(s) individually with a focus on their own childhood is often a helpful first move, since projection of unpleasant personal memories on to the child is a common underlying theme. This may have been made more likely by intercurrent depression which causes the parent(s) to brood on painful and unsatisfactory aspects of their life. Should a counselling approach to parents fail, consider a referral to a child psychiatrist.

Scapegoating

The child is seen, inappropriately, as the source of all the family's woes (and thus may be rejected). A whole family interview may allow the real causes of misery or failure to be identified. There is the problem that the child may act up to the label of troublemaker and be unwilling to give this up; however unrewarding it may seem to be, it is a role and way of behaving which he feels is demanded of him, and which out of loyalty to his family, he accepts. Formal family therapy is often indicated.

Discord

Open aggression, denigration and abusive disagreement between parents is an important source of psychological disturbance in their child, much more so than unspoken hostility. As a rough rule, open discord is most likely to be associated with antisocial behaviour. The child is upset, will copy adult behaviour and is unsupported and uncontained by inconsistent, irritable parents. Less commonly there can be threats to kill, commit suicide, abscond, etc., which are made during marital rows and overheard by a child who takes them literally, feels threatened and becomes insecure, anxious and clinging.

Triangulation

A marital dispute may not take the form of open confrontation between husband and wife but be routed through the child, arguments between the parents being focused on each other's handling of the child or their respective expectations of him. Thus what is essentially a marital problem is concealed behind complaints about the behaviour of the child. The child may collude in order to keep the peace but experience torn loyalties and consequent misery. He may act out the part of problem child, a role made easy by his confusion, especially if he is overtly asked to take sides with one parent against the other. Occasionally the child may be subtly encouraged by one parent to play the other one up, thus becoming a pawn in the contest between parents who have been unable to preserve an adequate boundary around their marriage, within which system the disagreement arises and needs to be resolved. Children should be kept out of marital disputes.

Displacement

A parent may find they have strong feelings, especially of resentment, towards a child. Although initially inexplicable, these may often be traced to feelings which should more properly be directed elsewhere. Thus a single mother may resent her small boy who presents an embodiment of the husband who deserted her. She may not be aware of this so that the simple question 'Does he remind you of anyone?' may be revealing.

Inconsistency

Parents who disagree between each other on handling or expectations or change their own stance from one minute to the next are likely to rear confused, anxious, angry or unsocialized children. It is the seriousness of the inconsistency which is the issue; most parents are somewhat inconsistent and it is frequently possible to blame inconsistency for behavioural problems merely because it is common. When inconsistency is obviously severe and undoubtedly contributing to a problem it is often quite difficult to correct, if only because many wildly inconsistent parents are confused and uncertain themselves. They may be depressed or have longstanding problems of personal inadequacy. Simple advice given to both parents as to specifically what they might do in particular instances is nevertheless a necessary starting point. A mere exhortation to 'be more consistent' rarely works.

Child mental health surveillance

A framework for assessment

There is no hard and fast line to be drawn between a child's physical health and his mental health. Opportunities arise during routine physical health care consultations for the appraisal of psychological development and prognostic signs. For any preschool child in the practice, a series of simple questions needs to be asked about his psychological welfare. They are couched in the male sex here because psychological developmental problems affect more boys than girls.

Are the parents competent?
In terms of their ability to protect the child, foster his socialization and self-esteem. *See* the section on family issues.

What is their attitude towards the child?
Positive or negative, overprotective, dismissive, etc.

What is the quality of the child's attachments?
Secure, insecure, avoidant or absent.

What is the overall quality of the relationship between child and parent?
Comfortable, tense, unstable, etc.

What is the child's temperament and how does it square with his parents' attitudes?
Easy, difficult, slow to warm up, boisterous, studious, sensitive, etc.

Are his parents mentally healthy?
Parental depression, personality disorder or alcohol abuse are risk factors for child mental health.

What is his capacity to learn?
General and specific cognitive development. Intelligence is a protective factor against the development of emotional and behavioural problems.

Is his language development satisfactory?
Developmental language delay may underlie aggressive outbursts or other behavioural problems; the child has to express himself in behaviour rather than words.

Is he learning appropriate ways of coping with challenges posed by development?
Such as separations, postponing gratification, having to give way to parental authority, etc. Many behavioural problems are manifestations of a failure to learn appropriate skills; the child is trying to solve a problem but using the wrong techniques.

Can he form and maintain friendships?
Poor peer relationships are a poor prognostic sign.

The answers to these questions can often be discovered by simple observation of parent and child during ordinary consultations and by a few conversational questions.
   Early, active intervention to solve behavioural problems is good preventive medicine.

Making sense of emotional and behavioural problems

Involvement in child health surveillance means that the general practitioner comes face-to-face with a host of questions and problems concerning small children's behavioural and emotional responses. This can be puzzling to the novice since such topics are scantily dealt with in most undergraduate and vocational training programmes.
   The first step in managing a child's emotional or behavioural problem is to obtain a description of the symptoms and their effect on the child and others. This should enable a decision to be made as to whether the complaint is about behaviour which is normal or abnormal for the child's age.

If you judge the child's behaviour and emotional state to be essentially **normal**, the question is why should the parent complain about it? Several possibilities exist:

- They may be ignorant (first child), misinformed, or apprehensive because of similar symptoms in another child (or the childhood of someone they know) who became a problem.
- The behaviour may touch a raw nerve with them, because it reminds them of part of their own experience or personality which they are uncomfortable or upset about.
- They may be concerned about something else and are using the problem presented as an excuse for a consultation.
- They could be overstressed or mentally unstable.

This means that it is necessary to go beyond a simple reassuring statement that the behavioural or emotional state is normal, to ask what concerns the parent most about the problem: does it remind them of anything, is there anything else that they are worried about, and how are they coping themselves?

For some symptoms such as babyish behaviour, clinging, misery or anxiety, the issue is also whether they can easily be understood as reactions to circumstances or whether they are so excessive or prolonged compared with what would be expected of an ordinary child that the reaction to adversity is abnormal. When the presenting feature is an emotional problem in a child over the age of about 4, it is useful to obtain the child's point of view and this may require a brief private interview. This can reveal private or secret sources of distress unknown to the accompanying parent as well as revealing the degree of inner emotional suffering.

Remember that the 'cause' of a problem is often a matrix of **predisposing, precipitating** and **perpetuating** aetiological factors. What originally caused a problem in a particular child may not be what is causing it to persist.

When the complaint is about abnormal behaviour which is episodic, consider an analysis which includes an account of the:

- **Antecedents**
- **Behaviour**
- **Consequences**

of a typical episode.

This should enable you to decide whether the child's response to general or particular circumstances is appropriate or excessive and what the impact upon the child is. Accordingly you can decide if the child's reaction is abnormal. If it is not, then the appropriate action is usually to inform the parent of the cause of the child's distress (provided that the child agrees) and suggest what they might do to alleviate it.

If an abnormality of behavioural or emotional reaction seems to be present then the next step is to estimate the prognosis. If this is thought to be good and the child is not suffering, then it may well be enough to **reassure** and offer a follow-up appointment which can be cancelled if no longer needed. Good prognostic pointers include:

- Good ability to get along with other children.
- Reasonable family (use common sense to judge).
- Good previous personality.

- An onset related to identified and reversible stress.
- Brief duration of problem.

Should you consider reassurance and an expectant approach to be insufficient, or if matters have not improved within a few weeks, then a more **active intervention** will be required. Approaches within the capacity of most primary care doctors include:

- Counselling parents.
- Counselling child.
- Simple behavioural programmes and contracts.
- Medication.

If this is inappropriate or insufficient, consider **referral** to another agency. Many problems involving preschool children or somatic complaints will be well dealt with in paediatric outpatients. If the local District clinical psychology service has an experienced child psychologist they will prove a most useful resource, especially with behavioural problems of young children. Departments of child psychiatry and child guidance clinics are often at their best with serious cases or complex family problems and see more school-age than preschool children. Very often, knowledge of local expertise outweighs any generalization as to which agency should deal with a child's psychological problem.

Child protection

> The focus of most work on child abuse is secondary prevention: to prevent further abuse occurring to a child who has already been abused. Primary prevention of abuse is more difficult and largely unevaluated. Adults' knowledge of the existence of reporting systems such as Childline and school-based programmes which teach children to say 'No' to sexual advances are thought to make a contribution towards preventing abuse happening in the first place.

Child abuse happens when social standards for the care and protection of children are betrayed. Such standards will inevitably vary with time as social expectations fluctuate. Thus there is now a consensus that **physical abuse** or non-accidental injury (NAI) may be defined as 'any non-accidental physical injury to a child which results in tissue injury'. Rates vary according to the age of the child and the severity of injury but lie between 0.3 and one per cent for preschool children.

Munchausen's syndrome by proxy (also called Meadow's syndrome) is an uncommon variant wherein a mother falsifies the account she provides about her child so that a factitious illness is created.

Child sex abuse (CSA) is harder to define but the following is widely employed: 'the involvement of dependent, developmentally immature children and adolescents in sexual activities that they do not fully comprehend, are unable to give informed consent to, and that violate the social taboos of family roles'. This will include a variety of acts: exposure, fondling, sexual intercourse and rape. Rates are very hard to define but lie between an estimated one per cent for serious sexual encounters to 10 per cent for all forms of abuse including exposure to pornography and verbal sexual overtures. Victims are more commonly girls and can be any age.

Emotional abuse essentially amounts to the use of threats, blackmail, verbal abuse, or other methods of intentionally inducing fear and crippling the child's self-esteem. The boundary between ordinary parental anger and abuse is hard to define but is transgressed if the child learns maladaptive behaviours or attitudes as a consequence; he has been psychologically scarred.

Non-organic failure to thrive is commonly referred to as the consequence of emotional neglect or a distortion of the parent–child relationship.

Neglect occurs when a parent fails to provide conditions or measures required for a child to develop physically, emotionally and socially, or when they fail to protect the child from avoidable suffering.

Many abused children suffer several forms of abuse so that there is some sense in discussing abuse generally. Deliberate, considered, sadistic abuse is even more serious than abuse occurring by default or on the spur of the moment.

Early detection of abuse is largely a matter of considering its possibility, either because the family presents certain characteristics or because the child exhibits certain patterns of injury, growth or behaviour.

Children with disabilities are at increased risk of being abused, particularly those with severe communication disorders. Presence of someone who the child trusts and who can understand their communication system (e.g. British Sign Language for the Deaf) may be essential for adequate assessment of suspected abuse.

Physical abuse

The following are predisposing factors for physical abuse:

Family any (not all) of the following:
- Socially isolated family or single unsupported parent.
- Materially disadvantaged with little privacy for individual members.
- Young parents.
- Lack of child-centred attitudes.
- Unreasonably ambitious or perfectionistic expectations of child.
- Parent abused themselves in childhood.
- Habitually violent household.
- Chaotic, multi-problem family.
- Male cohabitee who is not father of child.

Child
- Unwanted.
- Unacceptable (wrong gender, malformed, handicapped).
- Biologically unrelated to potentially abusing adult.
- Difficult temperament or perennially crying.

These interact with **precipitants**:
- Illness in child or parent.
- Social disaster such as eviction from home, loss of job, etc.
- Marital or child–parent dispute.
- Mental illness in parent.

Actual abuse can be identified according to **history**, **observation** and **examination**.

History

- A child alleges abuse.
- Unexplained delay between injury and presentation to medical services.
- Vague, inconsistent, varying account of how injury occurred.
- Story of injury incompatible with child's developmental status.
- History incompatible with findings.

Observation

- Parents' general manner towards child is negative.
- Parents respond to questions in an irritable or touchy way.
- Child handled inappropriately by parents: roughly, no eye-to-eye contact, no comforting when distressed, etc.
- Child appears exceptionally wary: 'frozen watchfulness' (this is rare).
- *Note* that child may cling and seek comfort from abusive parent.

Common situations

Parent brings the child to the doctor and BRUISES ARE FOUND:

- Why has the parent brought the child to you at this time?

- What explanation is given? Is it compatible with the shape, size and distribution of the bruises?

- How old are the bruises? A bruise that is going yellow is more than 24 hours old, but beyond this it is difficult to work out when a bruise was acquired. Be suspicious if the story is not compatible with the colour of the bruise.

- Are these bruises 'normal'?; bruises are particularly common on the shins and many children acquire other scattered bruises which cannot always be instantly explained. Certain patterns of bruising are more sinister: bruises on the face, black eyes, haematomas on the ear, a series of bruises on the back due to fingertip pressure, etc.

- Consider whether there could be a bleeding disorder. Bruises that occur in improbable sites such as the axilla, or that are palpable, or are developing very rapidly, are probably pathological. If uncertain, arrange for a paediatric opinion.

If you are still concerned about possible abuse:

- Express open concern for the bruises and say that you want someone else to look at them. For example: 'Mrs Jones, I am very concerned about John's bruises and I would like someone else to see them.'

- Don't lie to the parent; don't collude with the parent about e.g. 'being an easy bruiser'; if you do not feel that is a viable explanation.

- If your concern is initiated by repeated episodes of unexplained suspicious bruising, you can say: 'We can't let this go on, we have to look into it and find out why this is happening.'

Examination (the following are particularly suspicious):

- Head or eye injury (black eye, detached retina, subdural haematoma, skull fracture in a non-ambulant child).
- Long bone or rib fracture in a child under 2 years old.
- Burns with unusual outlines resulting from being held against hot object.
- Burns to buttocks, groin, or in glove-and-stocking distribution from part-immersion in hot water.
- Deep circular cigarette burns.
- Weals or abrasions with unusual configurations (e.g. crescentic, as inflicted by beating with loop flex).
- Bite marks.
- Finger and thumb grip marks or bruises especially on cheeks, ears, upper arms or back (from child being held and shaken).
- Injured lip and/or torn frenulum from ramming bottle or spoon into mouth, or forcing lips against teeth.
- Serious injuries of different ages.

Sexual abuse

Predisposing factors in intrafamilial child sexual abuse include:

- Mother who was herself sexually abused in childhood.
- Poor marital sexual relationship.
- Opportunity for perpetrator to abuse.

Unlike physical abuse which may be explosive, child sexual abuse is likely to be chronic and secret, presenting after it has been happening for years.

History

- The child may allege abuse. This should be taken seriously. It *may* be retracted later. A spontaneous, detailed, consistent account with an accompanying display of emotion is likely to be valid.
- Detailed knowledge of adult sexual practices is suspicious.
- The questions to be put to the child will vary with their age. Young children can be asked whether any grown-up has touched private parts of their body. Leading questions such as "Did Daddy . . ." should be avoided.
- Older girls can be asked straightforwardly whether any adult has interfered with them or touched parts of their bodies that they should not have done or that they did not want them to. It is wise to follow up this question with, 'Anyone at all? Even people at home?'

Particular behaviours should arouse suspicion (though usually have a more innocent explanation)

- Reluctance to remain alone with a particular adult.
- Repeated running away from home or reluctance to return home after school.
- Intentional overdose.

Observation

A chronically sexually abused child may be prematurely sexualized and behave in an adult sexual manner towards others.

Examination

Physical signs of sexual abuse are unusual but the following are mildly suspicious:

- Vaginitis or discharge.
- Recurrent dysuria.
- Enlarged vaginal opening.

The following are very suspicious:

- Bruising or laceration to vulva or anus.
- Sexually transmitted organisms in vagina or throat.
- Sexually transmitted disease.
- Pregnancy with no clearly identified father.

Common situations

A young child is brought to the doctor with SORENESS OF THE PERINEUM OR VAGINAL DISCHARGE—child abuse is not mentioned by the parent:

- These symptoms are very common in little girls, and are rarely due to child sexual abuse.

- Other causes are more likely: urinary infection, poor hygiene, infantile masturbation, pinworms, soap powder or bubble bath reactions, lichen planus, non-venereal infections, or the normal discharge which occurs as girls approach puberty.

- Foreign bodies in the vagina are rare, as are tumours, but unexplained bleeding before puberty usually merits specialist referral.

Nevertheless, the parents are likely to have thought about abuse; they will not mind being asked and may well expect questions like:

- 'Is it possible that someone might have interfered with the child—touching the private parts of the body?'

- 'Is there anything else you are concerned about?' or 'Has she said anything to you to make you feel worried?'

- Depending on the age of the child, you need to convey the message that it is OK to talk. By asking the questions mentioned above, you may make it easier for the child to talk to her mother at a later stage even if she does not do so at the time.

Emotional abuse and failure to thrive

Emotional abuse should be considered as a common cause of growth failure or developmental delay in very young children. In infancy, non-organic failure to thrive is a diagnosis which is conventionally made by exclusion of organic causes and will thus usually be made by a paediatrician.

Emotional abuse, in the form of verbal abuse, belittlement, mockery or cruel threats, may be witnessed directly. The parents may describe the child as always difficult and reveal grotesque disciplinary practices, including physical and sexual assault, that they appear to believe are necessary in order to control such a wayward child. Emotionally abused children thus tend to be either extremely compliant or aggressively defiant rather than anything intermediate.

Neglect with or without concomitant emotional abuse can cause short stature and mildly limited intellectual development in a school child. The parents or teachers may describe insatiable appetite, stealing and hoarding of food. They may have made arrangements for the child to eat alone. The child will show accelerated growth when removed from home, by admission to hospital for example. There may be additional behavioural problems: stealing from home, smearing faeces, intentional urination in inappropriate places, senseless destructiveness.

It is nearly always necessary to demonstrate that accelerated growth occurs when the child is removed from home before a Social Services Department will consider taking the case to court.

Management of a case of suspected child abuse

The prime concern is the welfare of the child and, if this conflicts with the needs of the parents, then the parents have to take second place.

Members of the primary care team such as the GP and health visitor are likely to know the preschool child and his family much better than any other professional, whereas the school child is probably best known by his teachers. They will often be the first to suspect abuse and will be intimately involved in the management of the child and his family.

In every Borough there should be agreed guidelines on the management of child abuse and these should be kept to hand and consulted in every case. The following plan of action should be considered in the light of such local advice.

How urgent?

If the possibility of abuse arises during a consultation, the urgency of subsequent action will depend on a number of factors.

- **The severity of the injury** and the need for immediate medical treatment. This must take priority.
- **The nature of the abuse**. Emotional abuse and non-organic failure to thrive do not require urgent action whereas NAI may do. Sexual abuse, if an acute episode, may require relatively urgent examination to obtain forensic material.
- **The age of the child**. A young child may be in more imminent danger than a school child.
- **The abuser**. If this is a member of the household, consideration should be given about whether or not the child can safely return home.
- **The informant**, if any. If a child makes an allegation of abuse it should be taken very seriously and it should be made obvious to the child that this is the case. If it appears, in the child's eyes, that nothing is happening the allegation may be retracted and an opportunity lost. This is especially important in suspected sexual abuse.

Common situations

A teenager discloses to the doctor that sexual abuse has occurred but 'wants it kept secret':

- One to one discussion with the teenager is important.

- Tell him/her that **privacy** is **OK** but that **secrets** like these are not healthy, therefore you will not be able to keep this secret and you will need to tell someone else. For a younger child in this situation, you can say 'some secrets are too big to keep'.

- It took a lot of courage to come to see you; you must now be seen to be taking urgent action, **even if** the abuse has been going on for years.

- Remember that the child **wants the abuse to stop**, that is why they have come to see you; therefore it is your moral duty to act on what she/he tells you.

- You can discuss the problem with social services and hand over further management to them, or you can ask them to arrange a meeting with you, in your premises, to discuss further action.

- The first task is to stop the abuse and protect the child: considerations of prosecution etc. are secondary. Many cases of abuse never go to Court.

- Try to minimize the inevitable harm done to the family following disclosure of sexual abuse, by making sure that the primary care team remains involved.

Unless the well-being of a child is in immediate danger it is rarely necessary to examine him without the consent of a parent or guardian. If a parent refuses to give consent, the child may still be examined if he is himself willing and mature enough to give consent. Alternatively, a Court Order may be sought. A child of sufficient understanding may refuse to be examined. Bearing in mind the likely antagonism that such a course of action could produce, it should never be undertaken lightly.

Whenever there is a significant suspicion of abuse the Social Services Department should be contacted after the treatment of any acute injuries has been carried out. The parents should be told of the immediate plans. Depending on the circumstances of the individual case and the strength of concern, the doctor should share his concerns with the parents. In some cases it may be appropriate to be absolutely frank, in others it may be better to say something such as 'I cannot explain these injuries and findings and I wish to seek further advice'. Doctors who suspect CSA but have little experience of dealing with it may find it difficult to raise the subject, yet the parent may be relieved to find that the doctor is prepared to discuss it.

Detailed notes of the examination and any discussions with the parents (and other professionals) should be made immediately and in your own records. Remember that such notes may be called in evidence before a court and that the parents may have access to them.

After discussion with the social worker, a number of courses of action are possible:

- **Examination by another doctor**. In the case of suspected sexual abuse, a detailed examination should be carried out only after a detailed history (investigative interview) has been taken. Young children should be interviewed by someone who has been specially trained. The examination should then be carried out by an approved doctor who may be a paediatrician, a specially trained forensic medical examiner or, occasionally, a gynaecologist. Repeated examinations often produce conflicting opinions (the signs may change over time) and are traumatic to the child. If emotional deprivation or non-organic failure to thrive are under consideration, a further expert opinion will be necessary.

  When non-accidental injury (NAI) is suspected, it may be helpful to have a further opinion when there is doubt as to the aetiology of the injuries.

- **Removal of the child to a safe place**. Rarely is it necessary to take a child away from its home. (Remember that social workers do not have a right of entry to a child's home—only police officers have this right.) If it is necessary to remove a child from its home, this should be arranged by a social worker. The Children Act, 1989, makes provision for a child to be assessed medically, against his parents' wishes, but without being removed from them (*see* p. 86).

- **Calling of a case conference**. The purpose of a case conference is for professionals to share information and to decide the most appropriate course of action in the child's best interests. Parents will almost always be invited for part of the conference, but professionals should always be given an opportunity to share information and concerns before the parents are brought in.

If abuse is confirmed, *and* the child is felt to be at continuing risk, the child's name will usually be put on the **Child Protection Register**. This confers no rights to any agency and has no legal standing. It does, however, signify the level of concern and usually results in continuous monitoring of the family.

As a result of the case conference, a plan for future management ('child protection plan') will be drawn up. If there are continuing worries about the family, the primary health care team will have an important role in supporting and monitoring the family. Minutes of the case conference should always be sent to the GP. These are confidential and should be filed in a secure place.

Many Social Services Departments circulate minutes to parents. If in doubt about what decision has been made in a particular case, the chairperson of the conference should be consulted.

Points to remember in the management of child abuse

- Do not panic.
- Keep local guidelines to hand along with details of how to contact the local Social Services Department.
- Take any allegation, especially by a child, seriously.
- Record full and accurate details of the history and examination. Make sure you date and time your notes. The parents will have access to your notes and they may be used in legal proceedings.

Common situations

The CHILD MAY ALREADY HAVE DISCLOSED DETAILS OF SEXUAL ABUSE TO THE MOTHER and the mother wants to know how to deal with the situation.

- Tell the mother to keep the child close to her so that the child feels secure. The mother may well feel disturbed and guilty about what has happened; her role as protector is important and you need to support her in this. The child has chosen to tell her and she must make the child feel protected and safe.

- The mother must demonstrate to the child that she is not angry with the child, or disgusted by what the child has told her.

- She must believe the child.

- She must not blame the child.

- Advise her to keep the child home from school for a few days. It is not necessary to tell the school anything at this stage; the child is 'under the doctor'.

- Tell the mother that it is your duty now to inform the social services, and that either you, the health visitor, the school nurse, or a senior social worker will be in touch with her to discuss what should be done next (if you don't know the exact procedure yourself).

- You may also need to tell her that the social services work with the police on such cases and that the police officers involved will be specially trained in dealing with children.

- Say that you have no authority to determine whether or not the police are involved.

- Throughout the intervention and follow-up procedures the mother should stay with the child.

- Promise to maintain your involvement in the case, but do not make any promises about what the outcome of the case might be.

- Consult with the Social Work Department at an early stage.
- Try to attend any case conferences, especially the first. The primary health care team often has unique information to offer. If unable to attend, send a written report or speak directly to the conference chairperson.
- Keep the key worker informed about any subsequent worries you may have about the family. If there is no key worker, inform the Area Social Services Department. Record all such contacts.
- If in doubt at any stage consult the Social Services Department, the Community Child Health Services or a Paediatrician.

The Children Act, 1989

This Act brings together most of the legislation covering the care and protection of children in England and Wales. It received the Royal Assent on 16th November 1989. Great efforts were made to ensure that it was written in such a way as to be comprehensible to professionals other than lawyers. The main provisions likely to affect doctors are as follows:

- **Emergency orders**. Anyone can apply for an **Emergency Protection Order** (EPO). A court will grant it, if it is satisfied that there is reasonable cause to believe that the child is likely to suffer significant harm if he is not removed to alternative accommodation or he does not remain in his current accommodation. If a Local Authority's enquiries about a child are being frustrated by lack of access, they may seek a **Child Assessment Order** (below).
  - The duration of the EPO is limited, in the first place, to 8 days. A single extension of 7 days may be granted.
  - The person obtaining the EPO has limited parental responsibility.
  - The court may ask for a medical and/or psychiatric examination against the wishes of the parents, but not against the wishes of the child.

  If there is serious cause for concern about the welfare of a child and the parents have not allowed the child to be assessed, a **Child Assessment Order** may be sought. This allows a child to be medically examined or assessed in any other way as directed by the court. The Order lasts for only 7 days from the agreed date and the child should only be removed from his home if it is necessary for a proper assessment. If a child is felt to be in immediate danger, an **Emergency Protection Order** is more appropriate.
- **Rules of evidence**. Since 10 March 1990, hearsay evidence may be allowed in civil proceedings in connection with the upbringing, maintenance or welfare of the child. Under the Criminal Justice Act (1991), children who are victims or witnesses of violent crime may give the main part of their evidence on video and will usually be cross-examined by a TV link to the courtroom.
- **Provision of accommodation to third party.** Where it appears to a local authority that a child is in danger if a third party remains in the child's place of residence, the authority is empowered to provide assistance to the third party to seek alternative accommodation. The assistance could be in kind. This is designed to reduce the instances where the child has to be removed from his home.
- **Adoption contact register**. In future the Registrar General will be required to maintain a register comprising adopted persons and relatives. An individual's name will only be entered on the register at their request. The Registrar General will then pass on to an adopted person (if at least 18 years old) who has registered with him, the name and address of any relative who has also registered. The address may be that of an intermediary. This should allow easier contact between adopted children and their natural relatives, but retaining confidentiality where required.
- **Disability register**. Each Local Authority is obliged to maintain a register of all children with disabilities. Parents may refuse to allow their child's name to be recorded on the register. While such refusal should not deny any resources to the child, the recording of the name gives a number of potential advantages, such as receiving mailings of information on various disorders, resources, welfare rights etc.

Children looked after

The law requires Social Service Departments to arrange medical examinations for children looked after ('in care') when they enter care, at six-monthly intervals until they are two years old and at yearly intervals thereafter. These medicals may be done by a paediatrician or a GP. A fee is payable when it is done by the GP.

The first examination of a pre-school child entering care needs to be thorough— these children may have missed out on medical care and routine checks, their parents may not have identified problems that would have been dealt with in other families, and their immunizations may be incomplete. In some cases considerable judgement is needed to decide whether a child is progressing as expected after removal from adverse circumstances—for instance, a child may be delayed in development partly because of deprivation and partly because he has a language disorder or hearing loss. Such cases probably should be dealt with by a paediatrician.

For older children, the value of annual medical examination is doubtful unless the child or young person has the opportunity to build a relationship on their own terms with their primary healthcare team, which might allow them to discuss their problems and their future. Thus the GP may be able to offer more appropriate care than a paediatrician.

Further reading

1. Home Office, DoH, DES, Welsh Office (1991) *Working Together Under the Children Act 1989: a Guide to Arrangements for Inter-agency Co-operation for the Protection of Children from Abuse.* HMSO, London.

2. DHSS (1988) *Child Protection: Guidance for Senior Nurses, Health Visitors and Midwives.* HMSO, London.

3. *The Medical Aspects of Child Abuse* (1989) A Report of the International Committee for Child Health of The Children's Research Fund. (Obtainable from The Children's Research Fund, 6 Castle Street, Liverpool L2 0NA.)

4. DHSS (1988) *Diagnosis of Child Sexual Abuse: Guidance for Doctors.* HMSO, London.

5. Meadow R, ed. (1989) *ABC of Child Abuse.* British Medical Journal, London.

6. *Child Abuse Trends in England and Wales 1983–1987.* (1989) NSPCC, London.

7. *An Introduction to The Children Act, 1989.* (1990) HMSO, London.

8. White R, Carr P and Lowe N (1990) *A Guide to The Children Act, 1989.* Butterworths, London.

9. Hobbs CJ, Hanks HGI and Wynne JM (1993) *Child Abuse and Neglect: a Clinician's Handbook.* Churchill Livingstone, Edinburgh.

10. Jones D and Ramchandani P (1999) *Child Sexual Abuse: informing practice from research.* Radcliffe Medical Press, Oxford.

CHAPTER 4

Tertiary prevention

Much can be done to alleviate the burden and distress of caring for a handicapped child, both in primary care teams and in specialist facilities.

Talking to the parents of a handicapped child

Parents are inevitably distressed when they hear that their child has some serious problem, but nevertheless the way they are told and the support they receive in the first days and weeks after the event do influence their ability to cope and to work with, rather than against, those who are trying to help.

When parents in your practice are faced with some major problem in their child, remember the following points which are emphasized by those who have been through the experience.

They want to be told:

- As soon as the doctor(s) are suspicious. If uncertain, say what you will do to resolve uncertainty (e.g. call consultant, arrange tests).

- In privacy.
- Without interruptions: hand your bleep/pager to someone else, divert the telephone.
- Both parents together, or with grandparent or friend if unsupported parent.
- Simply; not too much talking without a pause.
- At least twice. Arrange to see them again soon after the first explanation; parents do not take in what you say the first time.
- In writing as well as verbally. A written report and/or literature often helps.

Follow-up

Arrange a **follow-up visit** soon, by GP, health visitor, or social worker as appropriate. Invite parents to write down their questions in anticipation of this visit.

Offer to arrange contact with a **parent organization** or **individual parent**.

Do not burden the parents with your own solutions to their problems; **good counselling** is about helping people to find solutions that are right for them.

Listen to the **unspoken questions**. Will the child die? What is the life expectancy? Is it inherited? Fellow professionals (therapists, health visitors, etc.) are excellent at picking up these worries—listen to your colleagues who can tell you what the parents are really worried about.

Parents often want to know **what they can do** about the problem. Offer some practical help, e.g. Portage programme (home visiting programme which involves parent and adviser setting goals for the child and working out a teaching method to achieve them—derived from names of town in USA where it was devised).

Often parents want a **second opinion**. This is perfectly reasonable but it is important to choose someone who knows about the particular problem! If a paediatrician first broke the news to the parents, he/she will greatly appreciate a telephone call in this situation, so that the most constructive second opinion can be selected. If relationships with local services are damaged right at the outset, it will be difficult to offer optimal care for the child.

Deal with other **practical issues**, e.g. education, dental care, immunization, etc. when the parents want to discuss them.

Understand the concept of **bereavement reaction** (*see* Figure 4.1) and its relevance to handicap. But also be aware of the wide range of human response to grief; do not try to persuade the parents that they feel guilt when they do not! Do not expect them to exhibit these emotions in an orderly sequence. Having a handicapped child is compared to the death of a normal child and his replacement by one who is imperfect.

Special needs children

Any child suspected of having some disabling condition (e.g. cerebral palsy, learning disability, autism, serious vision or hearing defect, etc.) should normally be under the care of a **Child Development Centre** or **District Handicap Team**, where co-ordinated assessment and treatment can be undertaken. The aim is to help the child to make the most of his abilities, however severe the condition, and to help the family to come to terms with, and live with, their problems.

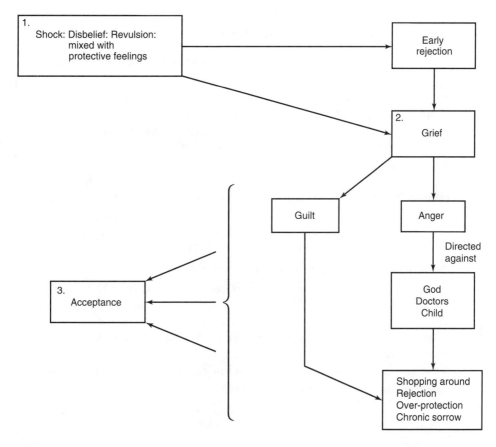

Figure 4.1. Understanding bereavement.

Minor medical conditions in special needs children can usually be dealt with by the GP as with any other child, although it may be harder to make a diagnosis if the child has difficulty in communicating.

Parents may ask about schooling. It is useful to know about the **Education Act, 1981**. This legislation was based on the Warnock Report of 1978. It emphasizes a child's needs rather than his diagnostic label; it calls on health authorities to notify the Education Department when they suspect that a child may have special educational needs, and also to tell the parents about the relevant voluntary organization; it gives the parents more say in their child's school placement; it encourages integration of handicapped children into mainstream school whenever possible.

Children with special needs undergo a **Full Assessment** (FA procedure) and a **Statement of Educational Needs** is made. These arrangements are the responsibility of the Local Education Authority.

One aim of a Child Development Centre is to provide a variety of services including information. The health visitor can contribute by visiting each family with a special needs child, to ensure that the parents receive all this information, at the appropriate time. A check-list is useful (*see* accompanying box).

Check-list for special needs children

Have you checked personal details; diagnosis; disability? Does child have or need a follow-up appointment?

- Do **you** understand the diagnosis? If necessary, check with SMO, community paediatrician or the child's consultant. Remember that in many conditions there are **additional complications** as well as those that are obvious when the diagnosis is first made.

- Do the parents understand who you are, and how you know that their child has a problem? As soon as possible, **explain about the local register of special needs children** as a means of improving services.

- Do they know **what is wrong** with the child? Do they have a **report in writing**, to show relatives, etc.? If the child is on medication, do they know what, how much and why? Have they a **record card**?

- Check whether a **hearing test** has been arranged.

- Do they want a referral to the Education Department? Explain about the Education Act and offer a leaflet if necessary. Describe **Portage home teaching programme**, if your District has one in operation. Do they want any **day-care** from either nursery school or social services nursery?

- Do they want any help from **social worker, psychologist, therapist, teacher, housing department** etc.?

- Do they want **books or leaflets** on the child's problem? If so, ask colleagues what is available (Child Development Centre may be able to help).

- Do they know about the **parent organization(s)** relevant to the child? If not, ask above sources. There is a society for almost every condition.

- Would they like to meet **another family** with similar problems? Same sources of information. Be careful; this can be very helpful but can be a disaster.

- **Financial help**: statutory allowances, Family Fund. Do **you** know the rules?

- Check that the child is getting **regular medical care** from consultant, including vision and hearing checks. Ask consultant if in doubt about what has been done. Don't neglect **routine surveillance** considerations: is the child growing, can he see and hear, any other worries? Remember that consultant clinics tend to concentrate on their particular specialty and can miss other health problems.

- Have they had **genetic advice**? If not, and they want it, check with consultant first. Have they had **dental advice**?

- If child is difficult and parental relationship is suffering, consider whether **respite care** would be useful. Some parents are upset about this suggestion; needs careful timing and handling.

Early intervention for developmental problems

It is difficult to prove that early intervention changes outcome in terms of the child's improved function, but it is certainly effective in reducing the impact of disabling conditions (tertiary prevention). Parents welcome guidance and support in the care of a child with a disability. For example **early physiotherapy and occupational therapy** do not cure physical defects such as cerebral palsy, but therapists often become the parents' main advisers on how to handle and care for the child.

Speech therapists may often confine themselves to assessment and monitoring in cases where a language delayed child is making satisfactory progress. Where the child appears to have a more serious problem, they may undertake more active treatment themselves or may refer the child to an educational facility such as a language unit.

Nurseries and nursery schools have a positive impact on the child's development, particularly if there is a well planned programme of activities and expert supervision.

Cot death (sudden infant death syndrome, SIDS, unexpected infant death)

One baby in every 600 live births dies unexpectedly for no obvious reason between the ages of 1 week and 2 years, 90 per cent before 8 months. In most cases, post mortem examination reveals no specific cause. Ideally all these post mortems should be done by a pathologist with paediatric training, since occasionally the death may be due to, for example, heart disease or metabolic disorders.

Although such tragedies are comparatively rare, in a group practice a cot death is likely to occur every 2–4 years. A GP may be called to the home or the baby rushed to the surgery; often the baby is taken directly to a hospital casualty department. GPs should ensure in advance that coroners, hospitals and medical deputizing services would inform the family doctor immediately of an unexpected infant death.

What to do if you have a 'cot death' in your practice

- As soon as you hear of the baby's death, **contact the family** to express sympathy, by a home visit if possible. Early support prevents later misunderstandings.
- Unless there is obvious injury, a history of illness or the parental attitude arouses suspicion, tell the parents it appears to be a cot death but that a **post mortem examination** will be necessary to establish the cause of death. If death remains unexplained, it may be registered as sudden infant death syndrome. Some parents want to see or hold their child after death is confirmed but before the body is taken to a mortuary.

- Explain the **coroner's duty**, the possibility of an inquest, and warn parents that they or relatives may be asked to identify the body. Advise the parents that they will be asked to make a statement to the coroner's officer or police, and that bedding may be taken for examination to help establish the cause of death. If necessary, give advice on registering the death and making funeral arrangements. The coroner's officer may need to know the parents' choice of burial or cremation.

- If considering offering parents a drug to alleviate the initial shock, it is known that many do not want anxiolytics or anti-depressants, but prefer something to **induce sleep**.

- If the mother was **breast-feeding**, give advice on suppression of lactation: prescribe medication and advise her to leave the breasts alone except to empty them once a day if an easy method is available.

- Take particular note of **siblings**. Remember that twin babies carry an extra risk of cot death and that a surviving twin may need hospitalization for observation. Give guidance on emotional needs of siblings, who may be neglected or over-protected; reassure parents that older children are not at risk. Do *not* advise parents to have another child as soon as possible.

- Advise parents of likely **grief reactions** such as aching arms, hearing the baby cry, distressing dreams, and strong positive or negative sexual feelings, but reassure them that they and other symptoms such as loss of appetite and sleeplessness are normal and temporary. Anger, sometimes directed towards the GP, guilt and self-blame, especially on the part of the mother, are common grief reactions for which the doctor should be prepared.

- Offer parents copies of the leaflet *Information for the Parents Following the Sudden and Unexpected Death of their Baby* and the address of The Foundation for the Study of Infant Deaths, 35 Belgrave Square, London SW1X 8QB; telephone 0171-235 1721 or 0171-235 0965. In addition to sponsoring medical research, the Foundation offers further support and information, and can put parents in touch with others who have suffered a similar bereavement.

- Make sure that parents have a **relative or close friend** very near them during the 48 hours after the death, and offer explanations to them and to the minister of religion. Make sure the family's health visitor and other members of the primary care team know of the baby's death and are prepared to give continued support.

- Arrange a subsequent meeting with the parents to **discuss the cause of death**. Make sure the coroner informs you of the initial and final post mortem findings and consult with the pathologist and/or paediatrician if any clarification is needed.

- There are some things you **should not say to the parents**: I know how you feel (you don't); you'll get over it (they won't); your other children will be a comfort (they might not be); you're young enough to have another baby (babies can't be replaced).

- **Warn** them that: their friends may avoid them and will certainly avoid talking about the baby who died; the baby's birthday and the anniversary of the baby's death will always be painful times.

- The **message from the primary care team** is: we care about you; we will listen; we will talk about your baby if and when you want to.

- Offer parents a **later interview with a paediatrician** both for themselves and the siblings. An independent opinion is mutually beneficial to the parents and GP, restoring parental confidence in the primary care team and sharing some of the load of counselling particularly concerning future children.
- Parents who have lost a baby unexpectedly will need extra attention and support with their **subsequent children** from their obstetrician, paediatrician, general practitioner and health visitor.

Reducing the risk of sudden infant death

- There are many causes of sudden or unexpected death in infancy and therefore there is no single prevention strategy.
- Some practices do reduce the risk and can be recommended, but even strict observance of these does not guarantee that a cot death will not happen. It is important for parents who have lost a baby through cot death to know this.
- Breastfeeding may offer some protection.
- Putting the baby to sleep in the supine position appears to reduce the risk. Some babies may need to be placed prone for medical reasons, on the advice of a paediatrician.
- Place the baby with the feet against the foot of the cot or crib, so that s/he cannot slide under the bedclothes.
- Smoking increases the risk of SID.
- The temperature of the baby's room should not be above 19°C.
- The head should not be covered; hands should be allowed movement (i.e. no swaddling).
- If the baby has to be put down to sleep in a warm room, use fewer blankets until the room is cooler.
- No more than 10–12 tog units of insulation are needed under normal circumstances; less in summer.
- Ill babies do not need extra clothing.
- Quilts and baby nests increase the risk of over-heating.
- Early recognition of symptoms of illness and treatment when needed.
- Frequent visits by a health visitor may reduce risk for susceptible babies.

Standard tog values

Vest	0.2	Sleeping suit	4
Babygro	1	Baby nest	4
Pyjamas	2	Sheet	0.2
Jumper, trousers	2	Old blanket	1.5
Cardigan	2	New blanket	2
Disposable nappy	1	Quilt (variable)	3–9

Care of next infant (CONI)

Parents who have suffered a cot death will inevitably be very anxious that subsequent children may die in the same way. The CONI (Care Of the Next Infant) scheme is designed to help allay this anxiety. It is organized by the Health Authority and involves the following:

- When the mother is pregnant with her next child and books at the maternity clinic, she is put in touch with her local co-ordinator.
- After delivery, she will be offered advice and support with a combination of frequent health visitor visits, regular weighing and/or an apnoea alarm.

There is no conclusive evidence that these measures do reduce the risk of a second unexpected death, but they undoubtedly reduce anxiety. Further details can be obtained from the community paediatrician, the Director of Nursing Services for health visiting, or the Foundation for the Study of Infant Deaths.

The expected death of a child

- The action to be taken should as far as possible be planned in advance by the paediatrician and/or GP. Should the child be hospitalized in the terminal stages? Are any tissues or organs needed for research purposes?

- Do not be afraid to use appropriate medications as for terminal care in adults.

- Do not assume that the parents will be relieved 'because it is all over'. This mistake is often made when the child is severely handicapped. There may be relief but also great sadness.

- If the child dies at home under your care, inform the paediatrician. Consider who else needs to know (e.g. if relevant, ensure that others are to be informed: playgroup, nursery, school etc.).

Further reading

Luben J (1989) Cot deaths. *Coping with Sudden Infant Death Syndrome.* Bedford Square Press (available from FSID).

Miscarriage, Stillbirth and Neonatal Death. (1991) Published by SANDS (Stillbirth and Neonatal Death Society): 28, Portland Place, London W1N 4DE. Tel: 0171-436 5881. (Covers both emotional and practical aspects of caring for parents who have lost an infant.)

PART 2

Putting the programme
into practice

Organizing the practice

Contents

In order to provide effective monitoring of the health of its children, a practice needs to devise a system to ensure that all children registered with the practice are reviewed at appropriate intervals. It is for the practice to decide at what intervals it wishes to review its children, who will be responsible, and whether it will be done by systematic call and recall, opportunistically or by a combination of both. They would be wise to seek advice from the doctor with responsibility for child health.[1] Before undertaking regular review of the practice children, it may be necessary to consider practice personnel, practice records and practice premises.

Organization

Team approach

If the child's parents are not to be confused, it is important that all members of the practice team are giving the same advice. This will obviously include health visitors and doctors, including those working in community clinics, and midwives. It will also need to be extended to the practice nurse and practice receptionists, and possibly include the school nurse (who might be consulted by a mother whilst collecting an older sibling from school), and nursery and playgroup leaders.

As there is a large body of people who could be consulted by a child's parents, it will be essential to devise a small number of statements about child care which can be printed and circulated. Priority areas will be different according to geography and social mix.

The first stage in setting up a programme of child health surveillance (CHS) will be a series of practice team meetings where important issues are discussed and a programme agreeable to all concerned is devised. As there may already be a Community Medical Officer undertaking the surveillance checks on the practice children, it would be advisable to involve him or her—or the Consultant in Community Paediatrics (CCP)—at an early stage.

Deciding the schedule of examinations

The practice team, together with the CCP, will need to decide the schedule of examinations, what important aspects need to be covered at each examination and who will undertake them.

Although practitioners are free to examine their registered children when they wish, it is sensible for them to comply with local policy in order to avoid confusion for parents and other practitioners when families move practice. Working outwith the District policy may compromise a GP's inclusion in the CHS register. This would obviously be financially detrimental for the practice.

The number of appointments required for routine CHS each year will depend on the extent to which the GP is personally involved in the various checks and procedures—this varies according to the policy laid down by individual Health Authorities. It is also important to allow sufficient time in the clinic to spend with children who are causing concern to their parents or the health visitor.

[1] This person may be a specialist in public health medicine, a Senior or Clinical Medical Officer, or a Consultant Community Paediatrician (CCP). As many Districts are now creating one or more posts for CCPs this term will be used in the rest of the chapter.

Identifying the child population

Whether the practice decides to monitor the registered children systematically or opportunistically, the target population needs defining in order that any who do not attend can be identified and followed appropriately.

A list of children registered with the practice can be obtained through the HA. This may not be up to date and will need checking. Practices may already have been keeping registers of transfers in and out of the practice and of babies born into the practice; others may keep an up-to-date age/sex register. These are both useful tools for creating the child register. Those practices which are computerized will have the easiest task. It will be essential to cross-check the register with the health visitor and the HA.

Registers

Keeping the register accurate is an important task and is probably best assigned to one member of the practice. There should be a practice protocol for new registrations, births and children leaving the list so that the responsible person is informed of all children joining and leaving the practice. If a computer is not used, a practice can set up a separate register of children, either using standard age/sex cards or customized cards which could include spaces for recording immunization and surveillance checks.

There may be a delay before a mother registers her new baby with the practice; cross-reference with maternity registers will be an important aspect of maintaining the child register. In addition to the good practice of ensuring that each child registered with the practice has regular assessments, the GP will need to identify those children for whom payment is received under the CHS list.

Each practitioner would expect to have between 20–30 children for each 12-month age band. It is therefore possible to record all children born in each month of each year on a separate sheet of paper. Next to the names, immunizations can be recorded as they are carried out, together with routine health checks. As each group of children will be together, any who default should be easily recognizable. The practice *must* be able to identify children who have failed to attend for immunization or for their specified checks. The practice will also need a system for ensuring that children born in the practice, or those joining the list, are offered CHS with the practice, and that the form is signed and sent to the HA.

Records

It is always important to keep clear and accurate records, to remind the doctor of his previous actions, to convey to other people what happened between doctor, child and parent, and to audit clinical activity. It is especially important to keep clear records when undertaking CHS, as with a team approach communication will be essential. The practice may decide to use an appropriately designed record card—either a District card or a custom-designed one. The record should have appropriate growth charts, and prompts for the necessary examinations. Additional prompts for health promotion and accident prevention are useful.

The introduction of parent-held records (p. 110) is likely to reduce the amount of extra space required for storage of CHS records. If the practice has an attached health visitor, or a close liaison with the health visitors in the neighbourhood, it will be necessary to negotiate whether separate health visiting records are to be maintained and how they can be made available to other staff who need to consult them.

Equipment

Before a practice can undertake regular checks on the registered children they will need to purchase essential equipment. This will include the following items.

General

- Scales suitable for weighing babies and toddlers.
- Height measuring device (p. 187).
- Mat for measuring length in babies (p. 125).
- Tape-measure for measuring head circumference.
- Auriscope.
- Ophthalmoscope.
- Pencil torch.
- Stethoscope.

The **hearing and vision testing equipment** should only be purchased after consulting with the Health Authority or CCP, because in some Districts this will be done by health visitors and the cost of equipment may be borne by the Authority.

Developmental review

A selection of toys such as:

- Plastic cup.
- Plastic spoon.
- Baby hair brush.
- Doll.
- Bed.
- Plastic toy animals.
- Small toy cars.
- Picture books.
- Thick crayons.
- Paper.

In addition, it is important to have available a few robust, safe and interesting toys suitable for babies and toddlers, to create a 'child-friendly' atmosphere in the surgery or clinic.

Premises

It is possible for child health checks to be undertaken during normal surgeries and indeed this may be unavoidable if a family has repeatedly missed appointments. However, a much more satisfactory service can be provided if a specified time is set aside for a child health clinic. This makes it easier to work alongside other health professionals such as the health visitor. As well as convenience for the practice team, it is helpful for the practice to think specifically about the registered children. It is also a good idea to avoid healthy children being in contact with unwell patients waiting to see the doctor.

The timing of a practice clinic is important. Many mothers will have older children at school or playschool. Knowledge of local social routines may help the practice to avoid arranging a clinic when mothers are likely to have other commitments.

In order to prevent toddlers from getting fractious if they are kept waiting, a selection of toys in the waiting room is welcome. The waiting area should be warm, particularly if it is here that mothers will be undressing their babies. Health education material should be displayed, ideally changing the theme each week or month to avoid boredom and torn posters. The display should be made relevant to children. This might be interspersed with a display of other interesting material, for instance local events. Care should be taken if free-standing display boards are used, to prevent accidents. If the practice has a video player and monitor, it may be possible to use suitable videos emphasizing health messages.

Immunization

Immunization is considered under practice organization in addition to the section devoted to it (p. 33). A well-organized practice should be able to achieve a very high uptake.

It is good practice to aim for a high uptake of immunization so that protection is provided for the practice population. Everyone who is likely to be concerned with immunization and children should be familiar with contraindications to immunization, of which these are very few (p. 38). Any misconceptions amongst practice personnel should be dispelled as parents will often seize any opportunity not to have their child immunized.

Accurate records should be kept and they should be regularly reviewed. Once a month is ideal so that children who have missed immunization can be recalled.

Paradoxically those children who are frequently in the surgery are those who are likely to miss immunization. If their records, their mother's records and their sibling's records are marked, the immunization can be given when they attend surgery with another member of the family. This will depend on observant and willing practice staff. A practice nurse who takes a pride in high immunization uptake will be an enormous asset to the practice.

Another group who have a low immunization uptake are those who are highly mobile. They are frequently seen in the surgery before their records arrive. It should be practice policy that as children are registered, they are seen by the practice nurse and information is collected about immunization status. The child's parent may have this information, but the practice nurse may need to telephone the previous general practitioner, health visitor or Health Authority.

As a last resort a practice may consider immunizing children in the home. If other measures are regularly undertaken this should rarely be necessary.

Gaining and maintaining skills in child health surveillance

Gaining skills

Caring for children registered with the practice is an essential part of general practice. The 1990 General Practice Contract identified the provision of a system of regular review of pre-school children as an additional item of service which attracted supplementary payment.

Each health authority (HA) maintains a list of general practitioners who are registered as able to provide CHS services. A practitioner may apply to be included on the list; they will be expected to meet the standards set by the HA. Most HAs respect the national guidelines, produced jointly by the Royal College of General Practitioners, the British Paediatric Association and the General Medical Services Committee.

The guidelines expect a practitioner to demonstrate competence in CHS and to have completed an approved training course. The Director of Postgraduate General Practice Education is responsible for approving training courses. Doctors sitting the MRCGP examination after 1991 have been required to produce a certificate of competence in CHS.

Maintaining skills

As in all aspects of medicine, health professionals will need to maintain and update their skills in CHS. Practice audits may identify areas where improvements could be made. These may be addressed through reading, lectures or group discussion. New developments such as the introduction of parent-held records or revised immunization schedules are likely to be included in the postgraduate education programme by the General Practice Tutor.

In addition to identifying their own educational needs, general practitioners need to consider the professional development of the practice staff and identify suitable training programmes with them. Aspects of CHS may be particularly suitable for in-practice multidisciplinary educational activity.

Reviewing performance

When a practice undertakes a new area of work there should be an in-built method for assessing the benefits and costs of the additional service. Preventive child health programmes are no exception. Records and registers should easily identify work-load, new problems diagnosed, referrals and use of secondary care, and immunization uptake.

It should be a simple task for a member of the practice staff to keep monthly records of the patients seen, those who defaulted, those who were referred for secondary care and those where a previously unidentified problem was found.

This type of performance review provides statistics which are vital for practice organization, although it might not reflect the more important aspects of the care provided.

It is equally important to review from time to time those abnormalities which were *not* identified during routine surveillance:

- How many children with a speech or hearing problem failed the first hearing test but subsequently passed and so were not followed up?
- How many school age children were referred for maldescent of the testicles? In how many was the diagnosis confirmed?
- Were any abnormalities missed because the health professional did not allow the parent sufficient time, or was not attentive to non-verbal behaviour?
- How many abnormalities were undetected because the health professional did not have adequate knowledge of normal and abnormal development?
- Equally, how much worry and unproductive investigations were generated by over-diagnosis?

Performance review will need to include review of clinical care, audit of records when abnormalities are detected late, and perhaps most importantly, observation of the doctor–patient interaction.

Further reading

1. Royal College of General Practitioners (1982) *Healthier Children–Thinking Prevention*. Report. RCGP, London.

2. The General Medical Services Committee of the British Medical Association and The Royal College of General Practitioners (1988) *Handbook of Preventative Care for Preschool Children*. RCGP, London.

3. Jones RVH *et al.* (1985) *Running a Practice*. Croom Helm, London.

Audit

Clinical audit is a study of some part of the structure, process or outcome of healthcare, carried out by those personally engaged in the activity concerned, to measure whether set objectives have been attained, and then assess the quality of the care delivered.

There is increasing pressure on all practitioners to become involved in audit of their work. Unfortunately, those areas which are the easiest to assess may yield the least benefits for the patient or the doctor. Audit is a term which has many different interpretations. It is often associated with the process of *external* auditors assessing the quality of a process.

It is perhaps easier to consider medical audit as both peer review and self-audit, rather than external audit. **Peer review** is the process of a group of doctors or other healthcare professionals undertaking similar work auditing together; **self-audit** is an individual assessment. Both should be enjoyable, educational and of benefit to the healthcare professionals and their patients.

Both peer review and self-audit involve the same critical stages. The difference, as the terms suggest, is that the objectives set by a group of practitioners are likely to incorporate several different views and will be a modification of many authors' work together with a practical overtone. However, working in a small group can have drawbacks; if criticism is insensitive it may lead to little modification of behaviour. The most successful clinical audit may be a combination of critical self-analysis and group discussion.

Choice of topic

If clinical audit is to be enjoyed and to be completed, the subject of the audit needs to be of interest; it needs to have well-defined limits so that it will be easy to complete; and it will be more effective if a topic is chosen which will allow change to take place relatively easily.

Donabedian first used the concept of structure, process and outcome:

- The **structure** of general practice includes the attributes of the doctor, the facilities available to him, and the administrative methods which are used to facilitate medical care.
- The **process** of general practice is most commonly chosen for audit, as it is the method by which care is delivered. The process can be evaluated by examining medical records or by observing the consultation.
- The **outcome** is the most difficult of the three to evaluate as there are many other factors which might modify outcome, such as socio-economic conditions. However, there are many outcome measures which can be used, such as the number of days which an asthmatic child misses from school which may evaluate the degree of control of the child's asthma.

Setting standards

It is important that as much as possible of our practice is based on established evidence. Before beginning an audit it is important to evaluate the evidence to identify the most effective practice, or where that is not possible to identify best practice. Many postgraduate education centres have the ability to undertake a literature search if it is necessary to identify the current evidence. Alternatively, as practices begin to work together in primary care groups, other practices may have already identified the most effective approach. Standards should be explicit and the evidence used should be relevant to general practice. This should ensure that the audit is clear and meets the expectations of general practice.

Information collection

If clinical audit is to succeed, collection of data needs to be as painless as possible. However, there is always a danger that data which are easy to collect are least relevant. Group discussion prior to data collection should prevent many hours spent retrieving irrelevant data. The choice of method will depend on the topic under consideration. A review of the records will depend on the quality of information recorded. Prospective studies allow ordered collection of data and this can be facilitated by using encounter sheets. The best results are often obtained when collection of data is delegated to a member of the practice staff.

Analysis of information

Once the data have been collected they need to be assimilated. A group may be able to determine the relevance of information in relation to the task of general practice.

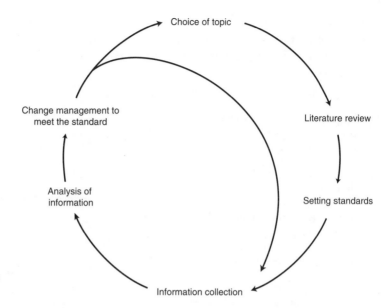

Figure 5.1. The audit cycle.

Review of the objectives

The analysis of the information collected should answer the question, 'What do I actually do?' and so allow an evaluation of the care provided. This may not match up with the objectives set at the outset, and consideration will need to be given as to whether the original objectives were appropriate or whether the standard of care provided was less than expected.

Either way, changes will result. If the original objectives were inappropriate they will need to be modified. If the actual care provided did not meet the standard then it is to be hoped that changes will be made in the practice to achieve the original objectives.

Monitoring the changes

Once deficiencies have been identified, further information needs to be collected to ensure that behaviour has changed to correct the imperfections.

Benefits

If clinical audit is to become part of everyday general practice, the benefit to the doctor and patient must outweigh the time involved in undertaking the audit.

If all the steps outlined (*see* Figure 5.1 for audit cycle) are completed, the audit should result in relevant and achievable standards of patient care. There can be no doubt that the audit will furnish the doctor with information concerning the delivery of care in his practice about which he had probably been previously unaware.

There are certain standards which we know we should strive to achieve, such as 'all children should be examined for congenital dislocation of the hips'. Unless we audit our work, we are unable to guarantee this standard of care.

Further reading

1. Sheldon MG (1982) *Medical Audit in General Practice*. Occasional Paper 20. RCGP, London.

2. Pendleton D, Schofield T and Marinker M (1986) *In Pursuit of Quality*. RCGP, London.

3. Baker R (1988) *Practice Assessment and Quality of Care*. Occasional Paper 39. RCGP, London.

4. Lawrence MS and Schofield T (1993) *Medical Audit in Primary Health Care*. OUP, Oxford.

5. Baker R and Presley P (1990) *The Practice Audit Plan*. Severn Faculty, RCGP, London.

The future

It is always difficult to anticipate future developments in medicine, but some changes can be predicted.

Multiprofessional approach

The trend towards multidisciplinary care is likely to continue. Children will benefit from the skill-mix found in most well developed primary health care teams.

Development of primary care

The National Health Service reforms have emphasized the importance of primary care. It is likely that most of the health care that our patients receive will be by the primary health care team, but this team will be enhanced to manage a wider range of conditions. There appears to be an increase in social and psychological illness created by the loss of the extended family and other sociological factors, and this is likely to result in an increased demand for more child psychological and social services, and an increase in special educational services. Practices may continue to commission psychology services from secondary care; the more innovative are likely to take on sessions within the practice, either from an outside resource or by arranging training for one of the existing members of the team.

Disease prevention and health promotion

Working with the educational bodies

Relationships on the education/health boundary will need to be strengthened, to provide the best possible services.

Caring for school children and adolescents

Responsibility for CHS is taken over by the school medical services on entry to school. Many general practitioners believe that their role should be extended into this age group. Although there may be organizational difficulties, the benefits of this group being monitored by their family doctor would be considerable. This would build on previous relationships and allow continued access to a doctor who is familiar with their previous illnesses and their family. Further training in educational medicine would be needed as well as effective communication with the school.

Immunization

Advances in immunization are likely to continue and the increase in foreign travel necessitates a more critical look at immunization for foreign countries.

A 'healthier' population

Our children are generally healthier, but, when serious illness is rarely encountered, it is difficult for a mother to view her child's illness in the context of the spectrum of disease. She will be likely to consult the medical profession more frequently for reassurance and explanation and requests for medical intervention may become more inappropriate.

Prenatal care and counselling

Few of our patients currently seek health advice before embarking on a pregnancy, but advances in genetics, prenatal diagnosis and treatment may lead to more demand for these services.

Consumerism or health needs assessment

Health services are much more responsive to consumer demand. This trend may force us to develop better methods of assessing health needs, so that the primary care team can respond to need, rather than the demands of the most articulate.

Technology

It is to be hoped that some technological developments will focus on communication, perhaps with a smart-card computerized record system, which could be read by the parents on a home computer.

Parent-held records

In many countries, a child's main surveillance record is held by the parents. A **personal child health record** (PCHR), endorsed by the Department of Health, has been introduced in the UK and is now widely available. National agreement has been reached on the format and content of this record, though local variations on content may be unavoidable (*see* Figure 5.2).

18 – 24 months review

This review is done by your Health Visitor or a Doctor. Below is a list of things you may want to discuss when you see them. However if you are worried about your child's health, growth or development you can contact your Health Visitor or Doctor at any time.

Circle 'Yes' or 'no' or 'not sure'.

Are you feeling well yourself?	Yes/no
Have you any worries about your child's behaviour?	Yes/no/not sure
Are you happy your child is growing normally?	Yes/no/not sure
Are you happy that your child hears normally?	Yes/no/not sure
Does your child understand when you talk to him/her?	Yes/no/not sure
Does your child talk normally?	Yes/no/not sure
Are you happy that your child's eyesight is normal?	Yes/no/not sure
Do you think your child has a squint?	Yes/no/not sure
Does your child walk and run normally?	Yes/no/not sure
Are you brushing your child's teeth regularly?	Yes/no
Are your child's immunizations up to date	Yes/no/not sure

(left margin: 18 – 24 months review)

Comment _____

Are all your household products stored out of reach or in a cupboard with a child-proof latch?	Do you keep your medicines and tablets in child-proof bottles and in a safe medicine cabinet?

Figure 5.2. A page from a personal child health record.

The personal child health record (PCHR) has the following advantages:

• It will make the information about the child's health and development easily accessible to the parents—the people who need it most. Thus it will be a useful vehicle for health education.

- It will accompany the child to nursery school, hospital appointments, school; and will go with him when he changes doctors or moves to another district.
- It will encourage openness between professionals and parents.
- It will simplify communication between professionals.
- It will reduce the existing duplication of records between community services, health visitors, GPs and other health services.

Experience to date is that parents welcome this system and are less likely to lose the record than are the professionals.

To be effective, the PCHR must be regarded as the main record. All professionals must use it.

- GPs and health visitors will need to record in their own notes that specified checks have been completed, but *details* of what was discussed should be recorded in the PCHR. The professional notes should be no more than a note of the contact *unless* some serious problem has emerged.
- Parents expect to be kept informed about any professional concerns about their child and do not appreciate secrecy. (In response to this frequently expressed view, it is the policy in many Child Development Centres and Paediatric Units to provide parents with a copy of all reports written about their child.)
- A more detailed file may need to be maintained for children with major problems, particularly those that have implications for community services. In particular this applies to children likely to require Full Assessment under the Education Act, 1981.
- All staff will be concerned about cases where there is a possibility of child neglect or abuse. Even in these difficult circumstances honesty with the parents will often prove to be the best policy. All staff must be aware that under *existing* legislation, parents can demand to see *any* of the records kept about them and their children; this includes social services records. Only in exceptional circumstances can this request be refused. In addition to these changes is the advice in *Working Together* that parents should be invited to case conferences held to consider suspected cases of child abuse or neglect. Staff will need further training in methods of recording information and communicating with parents in these situations.

The child health programme—ages for review

In thinking about child development it is useful to consider **five distinct stages:**

	AGE FOR REVIEW	
The **neonate**	Birth–8 weeks	(pp. 113–140)
The **supine infant** –	8 weeks–6 months	(pp. 141–150)
The **sitting baby** –	6–12 months	(pp. 151–178)
The **mobile toddler** –	12–24 months	(pp. 179–207)
The **communicating preschool child**	2–5 years	(pp. 209–266)

The approach to the examination is different at each stage. These stages also correspond to differing health education needs and accident prevention strategies.

Who should undertake these checks?

Each primary care team will need to decide for itself how the service is to be provided. The 8-week check includes a detailed physical examination and must be done by a doctor.

The checks for the sitting baby (6–12 months) and for the toddler (12–24 months) can be carried out by the health visitor; the small number of points which call for physical examination at these ages can be covered on an opportunistic basis, provided that they are completed within the wide time-limit suggested.

The preschool consultation includes a physical examination; this can be done at a special session with the health visitor, or on an opportunistic basis.

Use your time sensibly. Spend time with children whose development is causing concern, or whose parents have anxieties they want to discuss.

Arrange **more frequent contacts** if there is any cause for concern, but do not keep visiting or calling for repeat consultations without explaining the reasons to the parents. Parents soon learn that they are experiencing a different regime of surveillance from their friends and neighbours and they suspect (usually correctly) that the professionals are not being completely open about the reasons.

When thinking about the development or growth of premature babies, correct the age for gestation, i.e. a 9-month baby born 3 months premature should have the developmental level of a 6-month baby. But for immunization, do *not* correct the age for gestation; immunize according to actual age from birth (p. 38).

Birth to 8 weeks

Contents

This section is devoted to the care of the newborn infant and the first 8 weeks of life. It describes the changes in family structure which occur with the birth of a child and outlines the developmental abilities and progress of the infant. Detailed instructions are given for the examination of the infant at 8 weeks of age. The health education topics which need emphasis at this age are summarized.

Preparation for parenthood

In a stable relationship, pregnancy is a time of mental preparation for both partners, allowing them to consider how they will respond when there is a third member of the family and how they will cope with the inevitable changes in their life-style. If the relationship is under strain or breaks down, this phase of preparation may be disrupted.

Either or both partners may be ambivalent about the pregnancy. For example, they may be very young and immature, or they may have bad memories of their own childhood, or the woman may have planned the pregnancy in order to increase her chances of being re-housed (a common practice in some areas of the country). In such families there is a greater risk of difficulties in child-rearing which may present as behavioural disorder, neglect or even frank abuse.

There are increasing numbers of teenage single parents in the UK. It is naive to imagine that easier access to contraception would necessarily reduce the number of teenage pregnancies. Girls who have little prospect of academic success or of a satisfying career may see motherhood as a desirable option. These young mothers may have limited knowledge of child care, but nevertheless many are eager to make a success of the task and will benefit from advice and support if offered in an appropriate way.

Another increasingly common situation is where a successful high-achieving couple defer pregnancy because of career and financial considerations. These couples have very high expectations of their medical advisers; when they do have a child they may be exceptionally anxious about health or developmental problems.

For the mother, the transformation from competent business or professional person to nervous inexperienced mother of a small, demanding and apparently fragile infant can be quite disturbing.

The baby's life experiences will be shaped significantly by the family in which he grows up and it is not merely unwise, but potentially interfering and damaging, to consider child development in isolation from the family situation. (Yet this is precisely what happens when professionals carry out 'developmental assessments' in day nurseries without the parents being present and sometimes even without their consent.)

The role of antenatal classes

Antenatal classes, whether held by hospitals, health clinics, the National Childbirth Trust (NCT), or privately, offer education about pregnancy, delivery and parentcraft. The latter includes preparation for motherhood, a significant role-transition for first-time mothers. Intentionally or unintentionally the classes provide a peer group for new mothers, during pregnancy and afterwards. This can provide companionship and support for those mothers who would otherwise be socially isolated. Postnatal classes and postnatal support groups (run by most branches of the NCT) offer the same possibility.

Should a peer group become established, it can prove a valuable source of informal advice, particularly concerning minor problems of infant care. It can also offer the chance to share concerns and feelings provoked by child care without too much risk of criticism. In many ways it can replace, to some extent, the support offered by an extended family. This may help diminish the risk of depression supervening.

Child health clinics fulfil this function to some extent and this point should be considered when planning the introduction of children's clinics in a general practice.

Maternal bonding

Introduction

Early studies in the 1970s suggested that the first hours and days after birth were crucial to the developing relationship between mother and baby. Separations in this period might interfere with the new mother's feelings towards her baby so that she might never achieve a loving closeness to the baby and might subsequently abuse him.

The situation became confused by the practices advocated by Leboyer and his disciples. Birth was seen as a potential source of psychological trauma for the baby, the effects of which might persist throughout life. Babies therefore should be delivered in silence or to music, possibly underwater, and should be placed on the mother's belly as soon as possible in order to minimize the trauma of separation and emergence from the amniotic environment.

The beneficial result of all this was to humanize obstetric and neonatal care. Unfortunately there were adverse effects too. Novice mothers began to panic that they would not 'bond' to their babies. Some hospitals insisted on placing newborn babies to the breast or belly 'to help the bonding' even when both mother and baby were exhausted, or in the face of a squeamish mother's protestations that she would prefer her naked baby wrapped up in order to hold. Ordinary pain relief during labour became suspect because of fears that the baby's responsiveness to the mother would be diminished.

The facts are:

- The original studies on the adverse effects of neonatal separation have been repeated with better methodology but the original findings have not been confirmed.
- Most mothers whose babies are removed into incubators or are otherwise separated from them shortly after birth find that they develop normal feelings of love towards their babies.
- Some perfectly normal mothers do not feel anything special towards their new baby for several hours or even days but this does not usually matter. By the time several weeks have passed virtually all have discovered that they

love their babies. The few exceptions to this are usually under obvious stress, have developed post-partum depression, or did not want the baby in the first place.

- If there is a link between a failure of the mother to feel love towards her new baby and a subsequent risk of child abuse, this is extremely weak and only seems to apply when other stresses such as marital breakdown or eviction from housing occur.
- There is no obvious link between maternal 'bonding' and the development of attachments by the baby later on in the first year of life.
- Ambivalence about the pregnancy (unwanted child etc.) may only be fully evident when the baby is born and may be transferred to the baby. Whether this is dependent upon events in the first few days after childbirth is unclear.
- Some premature babies are insufficiently physically attractive to elicit feelings of love towards them as easily as a term baby might. The same is true for babies with physical handicaps. They may initially repel (facial deformity) or are unlikely to live long, in which case the parents may intentionally withhold affection to avoid bereavement should the baby not survive.
- Some babies are too exhausted following birth to be very responsive to their mothers. This may alarm the mother who perceives it as her fault.

It is doubtful whether any process in human development is so mechanical as to be switched on or off by different handling practices within a critical period of a few days. Life is more complicated than that and people more adaptable. Self-confidence, however, can be undermined. **Neonatal separations may achieve this for a minority of new mothers. Unwarranted hysteria about possible 'bonding' failure can do the same**.

Action

A mother who seems not to have any loving feelings towards her new baby is more worrying if she does not complain about the fact. One who is concerned that she has not 'bonded' will probably be all right.

Probably the most helpful thing to do is to undress the baby and carry out a neonatal physical examination, commenting on the baby's skills in looking, hearing, reaching, sucking and showing alarm. It is comparatively easy to show how the baby responds preferentially to the mother, looking towards her voice, gazing at her face, settling in her arms. The demonstration is essentially that the baby prefers his mother to the doctor and is a little person who can discriminate between and value different people.

While doing this, some careful questioning of the mother as to her perceptions of the baby may reveal anxieties or ambivalence which are blocking ordinary affection. Asking about sleeping and feeding will give some idea of handling and the extent of maternal exhaustion. Is the baby's father pulling his weight and what are his attitudes? Could this mother be depressed or overwhelmed with child care?

In most instances, the health visitor will be the appropriate professional to support the mother and monitor the development of her feelings towards the baby. A mother with a serious post-partum depression will need referral to a general psychiatrist.

Temperament

Temperament and personality influence the relationship between parent and child. Some parents, for example, may be very proud of a lusty, angry baby with a fierce temper, while others see this as an undesirable characteristic and would prefer a placid, peaceful infant.

A child's personality is not entirely the result of his upbringing. There are constitutional and inherited determinants of his style of behaviour which are usually referred to as **temperament**. Controversy continues as to which variables are best selected in order to describe and classify temperament and some uncertainty as to how great the contribution of inheritance is.

An influential project (the New York Longitudinal Study) proposed nine particular variables:

- Activity level.
- Regularity of biological functions (sleep, hunger etc.).
- Approach or withdrawal to novelty.
- Adaptability to altered situations.
- Threshold of responsiveness.
- Intensity of emotional reaction.
- Quality of general mood.
- Distractibility.
- Attention span or persistence.

This is not a list to be learned but an indication of what sorts of descriptive variables are used. Other studies have differed by introducing other variables such as fastidiousness, sociability or impulsiveness.

Temperament can change over time according to the child's experiences and may be particularly prone to change in the first year of life. Parental actions may intensify or ameliorate certain temperamental traits. It is crucial, however, to realize that temperament itself can shape parents' reactions. **The child plays an active part in shaping his environment which can then, in turn, shape him**. A highly active child may irritate his parents who react irritably and negatively, with the effect that his general mood is soured.

It follows from the above that a **goodness of fit** concept is important; the match between parents' expectations and personalities and their child's temperament. A poor fit leads to distress, even psychiatric disorder.

In the New York study, **three particular patterns of temperament** emerged which, taken together, accounted for about two-thirds of the children.

Easy
- Regular biological rhythm.
- Positive approaches to novel situations.
- Rapid positive adaptability to change.
- Predominantly sunny mood.
- Mild intensity of emotional reactions.

Slow-to-warm-up

- Negative.
- Withdrawing responses to novel situations.
- Slow adaptability.

Difficult

- Irregular negative.
- Withdrawing responses to novel situations.
- Slow to adapt to change.
- Predominantly negative mood (whines, grumbles, feels cheated).
- Intense emotional reactions.

The children with difficult temperaments (about 10 per cent of the sample) showed an increased risk of developing behavioural disorders later in childhood.

From a theoretical point of view, the importance of the concept is that it emphasizes the **interactive nature of social and emotional development**. The child is an active element and contributes to the quality of those interpersonal interactions which help shape his development.

From a clinical point of view, the principal implication is that some parents will need to be told that their child's difficult behaviour is not their fault and has not been caused by upbringing. It is the way he is and they need to devise ways of responding to it which are patient and positive. In other words, they must learn to respond to him as an individual in his own right and not to blame themselves for his difficult style. Nor should they become angry with him or themselves because of their failure to produce much change in him; change will be incremental and slow.

Normal development

Neonatal behaviour

For much of the day, the neonate is either asleep, or awake and restless or crying; but there are short periods when he is calm and wakeful, and there is intense eye contact between infant and parent. The visual acuity, although not at adult levels, is undoubtedly adequate for the infant to observe facial patterns and expressions.

The phenomenon of **'turn-taking behaviour'** which is a social activity that normally involves both vision and hearing, can be observed within the first few hours or days of life. The infant looks intently at the parent and this gaze is returned. When the parent makes sounds to the baby, he stills and listens. When the sounds stop, the baby vocalizes and increases his bodily movements. If these do not elicit a response from the parent, the baby may look puzzled, become distressed and even burst into tears. Sometimes a parent may suspect abnormality long before it is obvious to any professional, because they sense that the infant's responses and behavioural patterns are not normal.

Some young, inexperienced parents give adequate physical care and spend time with the baby but do not appreciate the importance of talking and playing with infants. They may complain of difficult behaviour, which in fact represents the baby's attempts to obtain the desired interactions.

In the blind infant, turn-taking behaviour can be developed only through the auditory channel and the eye contact component is lacking. If the parent does not appreciate these difficulties, there may be secondary handicaps due to lack of normal social interchanges.

Smiling and socialization. A social smile is observed in the majority of infants by 6 weeks of age and a delay of more than a week or two is unusual and worrying.

Vision and hearing. In these early months of life, the baby's sensory world is still very restricted, and he shows little interest in stimuli that are outside his immediate vicinity. By 3 months of age, he can accommodate for close vision and is acquiring a sense of depth and distance.

The newborn infant

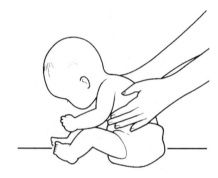

- The newborn infant presents with a mixture of floppiness of the head and neck and strong flexion of the limbs and trunk.
- When handled he requires support to his head and remains curled up in a bundle.
- He may be very insecure lying on his back, tending to startle easily.
- The baby may be happier laid in prone or on his side.

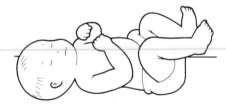

Supine

- Posture symmetrical.
- Flexion of all limbs and trunk.
- Unable to stretch his limbs.

Prone

- Flexed posture.
- Head turns to one side.
- Knees tucked under abdomen.
- Unable to raise head.

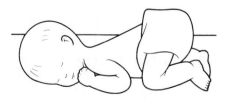

Reflex reactions

- **Grasp reflex**. If palm of hand stroked or traction applied to fingers, the infant will close his fingers tightly around the object.
- **Moro** (startle response). In response to a sudden stimulus of noise or movement the infant will fling his arms and legs wide and then draw them back into flexion.
- **Reflex walking**. If the infant's feet are placed against a firm surface he will move his legs as if walking.
- **Positive supporting response**. Reflex standing.
- **Sucking reflex**. If infant's mouth is stroked he will suck rhythmically.
- **Rooting reflex**. If cheek is stroked near mouth the infant will turn his head to suckle.

These reflexes are prominent in the early weeks of life. They disappear gradually and at a variable rate. The ease with which they can be elicited depends to some extent on the baby's state of arousal.

It is not necessary to insist on demonstrating these reflexes as part of the routine examination. Although neurological disorders affect them in various ways, there would always be other and more reliable signs.

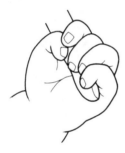

Grasp

- Hands held strongly fisted.

Age 1 month

- By 1 month the infant's limbs are more supple and movements more fluent.
- He is more tolerant of being handled and moved. He has a little movement of his head under voluntary control.

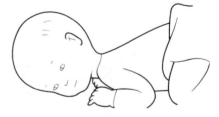

Supine

- Head usually turned to one side.
- Flexion in limbs still marked.
- Tendency to roll off back onto either side.
- Can partly extend arms and legs.

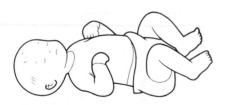

Prone

- Pelvis lies flatter.
- Legs more extended.
- Raises head briefly.
- Makes small movements with arms.

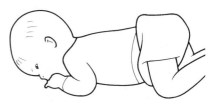

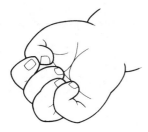

Grasp

- Hands less fisted.
- Finger movements seen.

Head control

- Held in sitting position balances head briefly.
- Head-lag when pulled to sitting position.
- In lying position turns head through arc to follow dangling object.

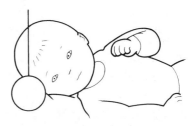

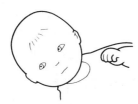

Age 2 months

- By 2 months the infant shows more spontaneous active movement.
- He is becoming happier in supine position.
- His postures are rarely symmetrical and he lies with his head turned to one side or the other.

Supine

- Lies flat on the supporting surface with pelvis and shoulders supported.
- Head adopts mid-position for only brief periods.
- Flexion of limbs decreasing—they rest in semi-flexion and can nearly extend fully actively.

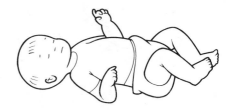

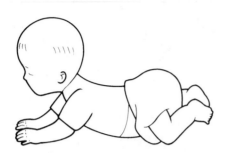

Prone

- Raises head to 45° and holds this posture for up to half a minute.
- Watches and follows toy placed about 22 cm from face.
- Follows this toy through small arc.
- Kicks with both legs alternately.
- Takes small amount of weight on forearms.

Grasp

- Hands open most of time.
- No longer grasps finger automatically.
- Hands may accidentally contact a toy in line of movement. This knocking action may be repeated if rewarded by sound or movement.

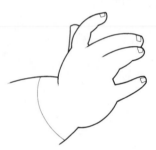

Being moved

- When held in mother's arms posture is more symmetrical.
- Shows a degree of head balance. This is not sustained or reliable.
- When dangled on his tummy (ventral suspension) his head does not flop but is held in line with body.
- Arms extend and abduct a little.
- Hips remain slightly flexed.

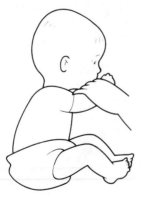

Standing

- Bounces gently on flexed knees.

Growth

Growth monitoring

Height, weight and head circumference (HC) follow a normal distribution curve. There is no exact cut-off point between normal and abnormal. **By definition 2 per cent (1 in 50) of children fall below the 2nd centile and 2 per cent above the 98th.**[1] In other words, in every classroom there are likely to be several children whose height, weight or head circumference is outside these limits. Only a small proportion of these children have any disease or abnormality. Of course, the further the measurement is from the 2nd or 98th centile, the greater the chance that the measurements reflect some disease process or other significant abnormality.

Weight

The regular weighing of babies may help in the detection of various disorders, but it is also capable of causing needless worry and unnecessary referrals. More importantly, since mothers like their babies to be weighed as a reassurance that the baby is well, weighing acts as an 'entrance ticket' to the clinic, an initial focus for the consultation which might be about feeding or growth, but could be about an entirely separate issue.

For these reasons, facilities for weighing should be readily available in the children's clinic, although it is doubtful whether mothers should be encouraged to continue regular weighing beyond 6 or 9 months unless some problem is suspected.

Scales need to be checked and calibrated at regular intervals. Ideally, nude weight should always be taken, but if this is impractical, for instance because the child is wearing a bandage or splint, the state of undress should be recorded. Weights may vary by several hundreds of grams depending on the contents of the stomach, bladder and bowels.

The weight should be plotted on the chart, after correcting for prematurity. Check whether the chart shows the years divided into tenths or sixths! If there is any question of abuse or neglect, the measure should be taken with extra care and double-checked. The entry on the growth chart should be dated and signed. It may one day be used as evidence in court.

Normal growth

The neonate may lose up to 10 per cent of body weight in the first week of life, although many lose less than this and some, particularly the small-for-gestational-age babies, do not lose at all. Birth weight is usually regained by the end of the second week and thereafter the average baby gains 150–200 g per week, doubling his birth weight by $4\frac{1}{2}$ to 5 months of age. The rate of weight gain progressively declines, so that birth weight is trebled just after the first birthday. In the whole of the second year, weight gain is between 2 and 3 kg. There is a relatively greater increase in length so that body proportions change.

---

[1] These centiles correspond roughly to the plus and minus 2 standard deviation levels (+/− 2 SDs).

Common problems

Whenever there is any concern about a baby's growth, the **length** should be monitored; increase in length is a far better long-term indicator of health than changes in weight.

- The baby's growth trajectory **may sometimes cross several centile lines** and this is not *necessarily* a cause for alarm. Birth weight does not reflect genetic growth potential but is more likely related to intrauterine environment. During the first year the growth pattern reflects the move to take up the genetic growth pattern. An upward move across the centiles may be a manifestation of catch-up growth in a baby who was small-for-dates; conversely, in the large baby of small parents, the weight may cross several centiles in a downwards direction.

- Slow weight gain dating from birth may be related to **intrauterine growth retardation**, perhaps associated with a dysmorphic syndrome, such as fetal alcohol syndrome, or it may be a sign of some underlying disorder of absorption, renal function, etc.

- **Transient failure to gain weight** or even temporary loss of weight are common phenomena and may be associated with minor illnesses or changes in care routines. Detection of these minor deviations in weight gain by regular weighing, as part of an intensive programme of support and home visiting for high-risk families, has been recommended by some authorities as a way of reducing the risk of unexpected sudden death in infancy, but this is not widely accepted.

- More serious degrees of **failure to thrive (FTT)** with the weight falling below the 3rd centile and continuing to deviate away from it, may require investigation. In the absence of other symptoms or signs, however, the yield of investigation is very small.

- The problem of **under-feeding at the breast** should be remembered in cases of poor weight gain, particulary in the first few months. While most babies will demand more milk if the supply at the breast is insufficient, some simply go to sleep soon after starting the feed, and this can deceive both mothers and professionals until the poor weight gain becomes obvious. Test weighing is unreliable because milk production varies so much between feeds.

- Sometimes poor weight gain is attributed to **inadequate mothering** and the baby gains weight rapidly in hospital or with a foster mother. This classic picture is relatively uncommon, and more often the baby's weight gain in hospital is also erratic, yet no specific cause is found.

  These babies with '**non-organic failure to thrive**' frequently, but not invariably, come from impoverished homes lacking physical comforts, emotional warmth and stability and sometimes adequate nutrition. Mealtimes are often accompanied by noise and disruption, and the child may be inadequately positioned so that he is not stable or comfortable and has no eye contact with the parent.

  The ability to manage foods that need chewing is sometimes impaired, though it is uncertain whether this is the cause or the result of the parents' failure to offer an age-appropriate diet. There may be impairment of gain in height and head circumference as well as in weight. Developmental progress is also affected in many cases and this becomes more obvious as the child grows older.

In addition to the parents' inadequacies, the child may contribute to its own deprivation by reason of unattractive temperament and behavioural patterns. Poor nutrition, in particular iron deficiency, may also play a part although lack of intake is certainly not the whole story.

It is a very demanding and skilled task to monitor such children in a way that ensures that the child's health needs are met, and social improvements are made where possible, without at the same time undermining the parents' confidence even further. Expert paediatric advice and close co-operation between social and medical services are essential.

- Mothers sometimes worry about **thin babies** but provided linear growth is satisfactory and the baby is otherwise well, thinness is very rarely a sign of serious disease.
- **Slow weight gain in the second year** is also a frequent cause of concern, and it may be useful to show the mother the growth chart and demonstrate how little weight is actually gained by the normal child in the second year.
- Professionals on the other hand, worry about **fat babies** in the belief that infant obesity is a predictor of adult obesity. In fact, this is not usually the case, and it is wrong to make mothers anxious because their babies are plump. Furthermore, babies have very clear ideas about how much food they want and it is not easy to reduce the intake. Only in the most extreme cases need any comment be made about overweight.

Always measure length when there is any doubt about growth, e.g. low birth weight, not thriving, parental concern. However, the **routine measurement of length** is of uncertain benefit.

A proper measuring device, such as the Rollametre, must be used (Figure 6.1); tapes on a sheet are not accurate! For the causes of abnormal growth, *see* p. 124.

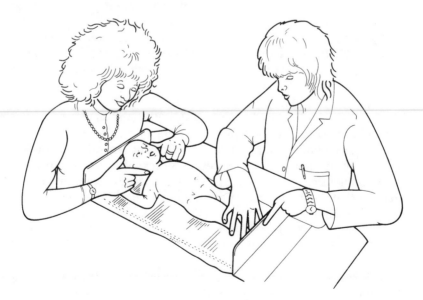

Figure 6.1. A simple device for measuring length in infancy.

Head circumference

The **head circumference** should be measured at or soon after birth. This measurement may be useful in the evaluation of neurological disorders discovered subsequently, to establish whether the disorder was pre-, peri- or postnatal in its origin. Neonatal head circumference should preferably not be taken on the first day as it may be increased by scalp oedema or decreased by moulding.

A second measurement should be taken at 8 weeks. There is no need to measure it routinely thereafter, but measure and plot it if there is any health or developmental problem or if the head looks large or small. Look at the shape of the head. Premature babies often have a rather long narrow head. **Plagiocephaly** (lop-sided head) is a common finding and is usually of no significance. Other peculiarities of head shape are more likely to be important and may be a sign of premature closure of the sutures. Feel for a prominent ridge along the suture lines and see if the fontanelle has closed. Refer if in doubt.

The head circumference should be measured using a plastic or metal tape; some paper tapes have sharp edges and cloth tapes stretch with use and become inaccurate. It is important to take the maximum circumference since this is the only repeatable reading. Many babies object to the procedure and it is wise to leave it until the end of the examination. The measurement is meaningless unless it is plotted on a chart.

Interpretation

Large heads. If the growth line is crossing the centile lines in an upwards direction, or if the measurement is above the 98th centile, measure the parents' heads, particularly the father's. A large head is commonly a familial feature; not only the size of the head but also its rate of growth can be increased.

Look for signs of **hydrocephalus** or **raised intracranial pressure**—separated sutures, full fontanelle, downward deviation of the eyes (sunset sign), squint and prominent veins on the forehead. If you are ever in doubt about the tension of the fontanelle, particularly if the baby is crying, sit the baby up and feel it again. If you are still uncertain, it is probably abnormal. Check for abnormal behaviour (crying, irritability, etc.) and developmental problems.

If these signs are absent and the baby is well, two more measurements at fortnightly intervals are permissible, but if doubt remains after that referral is mandatory. Hydrocephalus is not the only cause of cranial enlargement. With modern imaging techniques the problem of abnormal head enlargement is solved quickly and safely and there is no justification for repeated measurements spread over a period of months which leave parents in a state of chronic anxiety.

Never remark that the head is big or small without explaining exactly what you mean and how you intend to find out whether the fact is significant.

Abnormal enlargement of the head may occur at any age, and the head circumference should be measured and recorded in any child with a neurological or developmental problem.

Small heads. Microcephaly simply means a small head. **Pathological microcephaly** cannot be defined purely on the basis of size. Head circumference measurements below the 2nd centile do not necessarily imply abnormality. A head circumference which is *far* below the 2nd centile line is often associated with pathology and developmental or neurological disorder but this is not invariably the case. The measurement may be less significant if the baby is small or if one or other parent has a small head.

Microcephaly may be obvious at birth, or may occur as a result of severe perinatal or postnatal brain damage. These babies should be under specialist care so they should not present problems for primary care staff. Occasionally however, routine measurements of head circumference raise the possibility of microcephaly in the absence of any other feature. It is often difficult to decide how to deal with this situation and a telephone consultation with a paediatrician may be advisable.

Much anxiety is raised by suggesting that head growth might be abnormal but a decision must be taken either to dismiss the problem or to discuss the situation with the parents. They should be told that it may be necessary to observe the head growth for several months to decide whether the rate of growth is abnormally slow. Imaging techniques do not always help, and the developmental problems associated with mild degrees of microcephaly may not be apparent for 12 or 18 months.

Summary of the 8-week examination

- Check records up to date.
- PKU and thyroid results; sickle test?
- Review progress with parent(s) and health visitor.
- Maternal depression?
- Consider risk factors:
    - Vision and hearing defects
    - Other congenital or inherited conditions
    - Psychosocial problems.
- First impression:
    - Is the baby well?
    - Does he look healthy?
    - Is he growing?
- Look for:
    - Jaundice
    - Anaemia
    - Dysmorphic features—systematic inspection of head, face, neck, trunk, limbs, back, genitalia.
    - Tachypnoea and cyanosis
    - Genital abnormalities, especially undescended testes.
- Listen to the heart.
- Is development normal?:
    - Social and visual responsiveness
    - Smiling
    - Muscle tone and movements—handle the baby, lay him prone and supine.
- Check the hips.
- Measure and record the head circumference.
- Check for cataract with ophthalmoscope.

- Discuss health topics and immunization; sign up course of immunization and give first dose.
- Complete the Personal Child Health Record.

Clinical procedure

Every infant should be examined soon after birth and again at 8 weeks of age. Many GPs visit and examine the infant as soon as he is discharged from hospital. These routine examinations together produce a higher yield of abnormalities than at any other age and in addition they provide opportunities to discuss aspects of child care and family life with the parents.

Although the neonatal examination is performed by hospital staff, the trend towards very early discharge from postnatal wards (sometimes as early as 6 hours) means that primary care staff may sometimes undertake this important check themselves. This may also be necessary in GP obstetric units. The 8-week check will usually be done by the GP. In some practices it is done on the same occasion as the postnatal examination of the mother.

The procedures to be followed at the neonatal, post-discharge and the 8-week examinations have much in common and will be described together, except where particular differences are emphasized.

History and evaluation

- Make sure the baby's records are up to date.
- Any special problems noted on hospital discharge summary?
- Are the results of PKU and hypothyroidism screening tests available? These are occasionally overlooked, even in the best regulated systems. This is particularly likely to occur with babies who have other medical problems in the neonatal period.
- Does your Health Authority provide a haemoglobinopathy screening service for ethnic minorities? If so, have you got the result? If not, should you arrange the test yourself? Early diagnosis of sickle-cell disease can be life-saving.

Ask

- How is the baby? How are you coping? Any special worries?
- Is feeding causing any problems?
- Are you getting adequate sleep?
- Any worries about general health, growth, responsiveness, vision or hearing?
- Was the baby premature? If so, correct the chronological age by the appropriate number of weeks before interpreting your findings. (*But* immunizations should be given in accordance with uncorrected chronological age.)

Maternal depression

- Within 2 weeks of giving birth about two-thirds of all women experience an instability of mood with ready weepiness. This **maternity or baby blues**, is innocent and passes within hours or days.

- Rarely an **acute puerperal psychosis** develops, nearly always in the first 2 weeks postpartum. The patient is clearly severely disturbed, usually with a mixture of affective and schizophrenic features and a degree of disorientation. Response to treatment is good, as is prognosis, but because of the implications for child safety, this is a psychiatric emergency requiring admission to hospital.

- Mothers with babies and young children are particularly vulnerable to **depression with a large reactive component**. The reasons for this are incompletely understood but may include:

- Loss of previous social contact and support (friends, job, etc.).

- Continuing reduced social contact because of baby's demands.

- General exhaustion and lack of sleep.

- Husband spending more time away from home in evenings.

- Friction with husband, in-laws and parents.

- Feelings of helplessness if a combination of difficult baby and poor parenting skills, especially those requiring organization.

This latter condition—simple depression—can arise at any time during the child's early life and may have adverse effects on the child's development. Many depressed mothers are both irritable and inert so that the child becomes aggressive, understimulated and uncontrolled. There is a risk of child abuse and marital breakdown.

All depressed people should be asked about suicidal intent and a psychiatrist involved if necessary.

The management is, in the first place, two-pronged:

- To attempt to correct situational factors which are thought to be causal.

- To minimize stress on the mother.

There is no single formula but the following are common manoeuvres:

- Individual support from a health visitor or social worker (practical advice is often better received than counselling).

- Help with taking the baby out: friends, relatives or day nursery.

- Assistance with building a social network. If a self-help group such as Newpin is available locally, this is invaluable.

- Antidepressive drugs are commonly prescribed but their role is poorly evaluated. They are thought most likely to succeed when biological symptoms (sleep, appetite and weight) are disturbed. There are no grounds for preferring any one over another but the modern derivatives of the tricyclics or SSRIs are usually favoured. If effective, they should be taken for 6 months.

Risk factors for child neglect and abuse (*see also* p. 78)

- Very young parent(s).
- Lack of social support network.
- History of deprivation or abuse in parent's own childhood.
- Parent(s) attended special school.
- Handling problems: baby held at arm's length, lack of eye contact, no evidence of pleasure in the baby, rough or careless handling.
- Disparaging remarks about baby's appearance, behaviour, responsiveness or sex.
- Failure to thrive.
- Failure to seek medical advice when appropriate.
- Abnormal baby—prematurity, handicap, chronic illness, etc.
- Baby with difficult temperament.
- History of previous unexplained infant death in suspicious circumstances.
- Arrival in household of new partner who is not the baby's natural parent.
- Substance abuse.
- Family history of violence.
- Parents lacking basic knowledge of child development.

Parents who *express* a fear of hurting the baby should be taken seriously—but do not create a sense of panic or over-react! Discuss the reasons; what support they have and need; help them plan what to do when they feel under stress.

Look for

- Evidence of additional stress on the family: bad housing, financial problems, relationship under strain.
- Maternal depression—*very* common (*see* p. 129). Ask the mother how she feels herself, how are her spirits, is she enjoying the baby?

Consider

If the baby is in a 'high-risk' category for:
- Vision defects (p. 139, 174).
- Hearing defects (p. 138, 169).
- Any other congenital disorder.
- Inadequate care, abuse or neglect (*see box* above).

Check

If you are responsible for neonatal examinations, check whether the baby needs vitamin K, according to local policy.

The vitamin K story and haemorrhagic disease of the newborn (HDN)

- Newborn infants have very low levels of vitamin K, which is needed for normal clotting.

- In the newborn, impaired clotting can lead to haemorrhage from the umbilical cord, gums, bowel, or from surgical procedures like circumcision. There is also a risk of serious bleeding into the brain. This can occur at any time in the first few months of life.

- Modern formula feeds contain vitamin K. Breast-fed babies are more likely to be vitamin K deficient.

- Vitamin K has been given i.m. for many years to counter the risk of bleeding. It was suggested in 1990 that this might increase the risk of childhood cancers. The finding was highly controversial but pending further research the use of smaller doses, by the oral route, was suggested as a precautionary measure. *No confirmatory evidence has been found in several further studies.*

Policy for giving vitamin K is based on the following points:

- The risk of HDN is increased in babies who are sick; born prematurely; delivered by forceps or ventouse; very bruised; born to mothers on anti-coagulants, anti-convulsants or anti-tuberculous therapy. These babies should receive vitamin K by i.m. injection.

- Intramuscular injection of vitamin K offers the best protection against HDN for *all* babies.

- For parents who do not want i.m. injections for their baby, the alternative is oral vitamin K; this must be given soon after birth to prevent the early form of HDN.

- Babies fully or mainly formula fed do not need any further doses of vitamin K.

- Babies who are exclusively breastfed need extra vitamin K if they do not receive the i.m. injection at birth. This is available as Konakion injection (unlicensed) or Konakion MM paediatric (licensed) and should be given at birth, one week and four weeks. *This is very important. Forgetting can have disastrous consequences—brain haemorrhage or even death.*

- Parents have been very worried by the vitamin K saga, so …

MAKE SURE MOTHERS KNOW THAT: the cancer risk has not been confirmed in any other research study; the hazards of vitamin K deficiency bleeding and the effectiveness of vitamin K prophylaxis are beyond doubt.

Examination

This is described in three sections:

- General examination, including check for dysmorphic features.
- Examination of individual systems.
- Developmental examination.

General examination

- If the baby is quiet or asleep, do not ask the mother to undress him until you have listened to the heart and chest; this can usually be done by loosening the top clothing.
- While the baby is being undressed, look at the baby's general state of health, nutrition and care. The baby should be weighed while undressed and the weight plotted on the chart.

Check the following

Prolonged jaundice can be due to cholestatic liver disease, urinary tract infection, haemolysis or other serious conditions. However, jaundice in the early weeks of life is very common; it is often still present at 14 days of age. In formula fed babies it rarely persists much beyond this age but about 10% of breastfed babies are visibly jaundiced at 28 days and in many it persists for several more weeks. Breast milk related jaundice is benign and the baby is entirely well. The cause is unknown. Only a minority of these come to the attention of health professionals.

It is not feasible or desirable to investigate all jaundiced babies, but the following features require *immediate* referral to a paediatrician: any formula fed baby with persisting jaundice; any baby who is unwell or not thriving; unexplained bruising (which can be an early sign of liver disease); pale, creamy or clay coloured stools; urine which is yellow or orange rather than the usual almost colourless urine seen in babies; clinical suspicion of anaemia; itching (extremely rare!).

Dysmorphic features

The term 'dysmorphic features' includes any anomaly of structure which results in an abnormal appearance of any part of the body. They may result from chromosome or single gene defects, adverse intrauterine influences such as alcohol, or from a wide variety of as yet unspecified causes.

Some dysmorphic features are regarded as minor and are of little significance, for example clinodactyly (incurved little finger).

With a little practice, it is possible to carry out a systematic examination for dysmorphic features in a very short time, and you should not be put off by the long list of abnormalities which is given below. Experience is required to know whether a particular dysmorphic feature is likely to be significant and, if so, what diagnoses need to be considered. Always check whether the feature is a family characteristic! If still in doubt, telephone a paediatrician for advice.

- Begin your inspection by looking at the baby's **overall appearance**. If you feel that the child does look dysmorphic, try to decide what specific features give that impression. Check to see whether these are also present in one or other parent.

- Examine the **face** carefully. The **ears** may be regarded as low set if all of the pinna is below the level of the angle of the orbit. They may be underdeveloped, of an abnormal shape, or protruding excessively ('bat ears'). Make sure that the **auditory canal** is patent, but there is no need to spend time trying to visualize the eardrums unless the baby is ill.

  The **nose** may be uptilted so that the nostrils face forwards; this may be significant if combined with other dysmorphic features. A swelling at the root of the **nose** may look like an innocent cyst, but it could be an encephalocoel and may merit a neurosurgical opinion. The presence of **teeth** at birth may denote one of several dysmorphic syndromes. **Cleft lip or palate** should, of course, be referred promptly to the plastic surgeon.

- Look at the **shape of the head** and check the **fontanelles**. The posterior is often very small and may be hardly palpable by 6 weeks; the anterior usually closes by 18 months. The fontanelles vary considerably in size, and the variations are rarely significant unless the head is of abnormal size or shape. A long, thin head is characteristic of very premature babies, but otherwise may suggest premature fusion of the sagittal suture. A tower shaped head may occur with premature fusion of the coronal suture.

- Check the **eyes and vision** (p. 139).

- An unduly **short neck**, with or without webbing, may be found in Turner's syndrome or Klippel–Feil syndrome. An **underdeveloped lower jaw** is found in Pierre–Robin syndrome (respiratory and feeding difficulties). A sterno-mastoid tumour[1] is a swelling in the muscle, associated with some restriction of movement. Gentle stretching exercises may be helpful and can be demonstrated by a physiotherapist.

- Look at the **limbs**. Unusually short limbs occur in various skeletal dysplasias. **Asymmetry** in the size of the limbs, or indeed between the entire left and right sides of the body, is found in a number of syndromes.

- Examine the **hands**. Accessory digits, single palmar creases and clinodactyly are generally of no significance, unless associated with other findings.

- Look at the **lower limbs**. Under-development or wasting of one leg or calf may be the result of spinal dysraphism (see below). Deformities of the **feet** are common in the neonate. The commonest is positional talipes, in which the abnormal position of the foot can be corrected passively. Any other abnormality of the feet requires orthopaedic advice. Unexplained non-pitting **oedema** of the feet in the neonate can be a sign of Turner's syndrome.

- Examine the **skin**. Excessive laxity of the skin, so that it can be picked up in folds, suggests a congenital connective tissue disorder. Pink capillary naevi on the forehead or back of the neck are common and generally of no significance. A naevus distributed in the territory of the trigeminal nerve, however, suggests the Sturge–Weber syndrome; it may be small or extensive.

- **Strawberry naevi** which are invisible or tiny at birth and grow rapidly in infancy, are the cause of considerable alarm and distress to parents but are nevertheless benign and should usually be left alone. One exception to this

---

[1] Explain to the mother that the word 'tumour' is old-fashioned but still used. The lump is actually a fibrous scar and is *not* malignant or serious.

rule is when the strawberry naevus occurs on the eyelid or margin of the orbit as it may then obscure vision and cause amblyopia.

- Look for evidence of **occult spinal dysraphism** (spina bifida occulta). A tiny dimple whose floor is easily visible is commonly found in the cleft between the buttocks and is of no importance. There are, however, a number of other cutaneous findings over the mid-line of the spine, particularly in the **lumbosacral region** which, though apparently trivial in themselves, may indicate the presence of a potentially serious anomaly of the spinal cord. Look carefully for a tuft of hair which may look like a pony tail; a deep sinus or pits whose floor is not visible; a capillary naevus; a lipoma or dermoid; a Z-shaped deviation in the buttock cleft.

  If any of these are present the child should be referred to a paediatrician or paediatric neurosurgeon.

- Inspect the **genitalia**. Note and record whether both **testes** are fully descended into the scrotal sac. If they are, they are extremely unlikely to

---

Circumcision

Circumcision may be recommended for:

- Religious reasons.

- Public health reasons: possible reduction in risks of cancer of the penis, cancer of the cervix in sexual partners, urinary tract infection. The evidence of benefit in each case is equivocal.

- Non-retractile foreskin is NOT an indication. At birth, 4% of babies have retractile foreskin. With age, the foreskin becomes retractile without medical help. In boys who have had no medical or surgical intervention, at age 5, 90% have retractile foreskins; at age 17, only 1%. Preputial adhesions usually resolve without treatment. They may be *caused* by misguided attempts to retract the foreskin.

- Pushing the foreskin towards the baby shows a small orifice which can alarm the mother; if the foreskin is pulled towards the observer, the orifice is demonstrated to be adequate.

- Ballooning of the foreskin on micturition is *not* an indication, unless it is causing urinary dribbling.

- In 3–5 year olds, a tight rim proximal to the meatal orifice can often be loosened by application of 0.5% hydrocortisone cream twice daily for a few days.

- Recurrent balanoposthitis may be an indication but one attack is not. Chronic balanitis, true phimosis (with scarring of the foreskin) and meatal stenosis need specialist attention.

- Proteus infection is a definite indication for circumcision (after investigation of the urinary tract).

NB: Circumcision does have a morbidity and even mortality, although these are very low.

ascend subsequently. Testes which are not *completely* descended should be re-examined at 6–9 months and the child should be referred if doubt remains.
- Check for **hypospadias**. In the female, check for fusion of the labia and any anatomical abnormality. In both sexes confirm that the anus is patent. You may be asked about circumcision (*see box* p. 134).

Examination of individual systems

- Examine the **cardiovascular system**. The most important features of serious congenital heart disease in the first few weeks of life are **persisting tachypnoea, cyanosis, tiredness with feeding and failure to thrive**. Serious heart disease can be present even when there is no audible murmur.

    Check the quality and rate of the radial or brachial pulse, palpate the femorals or the dorsalis pedis pulse, feel for right and left ventricular enlargement and thrills. Auscultate for murmurs. If you hear a murmur, listen over the back as well as the front of the chest; some murmurs are louder posteriorly (e.g. patent ductus).

    If you suspect congenital heart disease in the first few weeks of life, consider the urgency of the referral. It is **urgent** if the baby is cyanosed or tachypnoeic. Symptomatic infants with congenital heart lesions can deteriorate very rapidly.

- **Examine the chest**. Look for **tachypnoea** and recession. Some babies who are slightly wheezy do show some tachypnoea but are otherwise obviously well. A **persistent cough in early infancy** is unusual and is likely to indicate some serious problem such as cystic fibrosis.

- **Examine the abdomen**. In the neonate, check whether there are one or two umbilical arteries. A single artery without other abnormalities is usually of no significance but it should be recorded.

    Small umbilical **granulomas** are common. The traditional treatment is to touch them with a silver nitrate stick, having first protected the surrounding skin with Vaseline. Warn the mother not to leave the baby in wet nappies for long periods as an unpleasant skin reaction may result.

    Check for enlargement of the **liver** and **kidneys**. The liver edge may be felt up to 2 cm below the costal margin. A palpable spleen tip is commonly found in infancy and childhood and is seldom of any significance unless greatly enlarged.

Developmental examination

- **Look first at social behaviour**. Observe the eye contact between baby and parent. Note whether he **visually tracks** the parent's face if they move in front of him. This can usually be demonstrated well before 8 weeks, but it cannot always be seen in the clinic, and some babies do seem to show a delay in the maturation of visual function. If in doubt however, get an expert opinion.
- Ask if the baby is **smiling**; this is usually observed by 6 weeks of age or very soon afterwards. Delay of more than a week or so in this milestone is worrying.
- **Ask the parents** about the baby's **hearing and vision**, but do not attempt any formal test at this stage.
- Look at **motor development**. Observe the resting posture while the baby is in the parent's arms. **Hold the child yourself** in order to assess the muscle tone

and then place him supine on the couch. Note the amount, symmetry and pattern of spontaneous movements. Hold the baby's hands and gently **pull** him to the **sitting** position, then lower him to supine again, noting the tone of the muscles and the amount of **head control**.

- Place the baby in the **prone** position and observe the posture of the head and any attempt to lift the head and shoulders clear of the couch.
- Do not try to demonstrate the Moro response unless you already suspect asymmetry of arm movement, which can usually be observed just as accurately by watching spontaneous activity.
- Do not worry about the other 'primitive reflexes'; they are only unequivocally abnormal when other easier signs of developmental problems are also present. Do not routinely test the tendon reflexes or look for ankle clonus.
- Lastly, check the **hips** and measure the **head circumference**.

Interpretation of developmental observations

Delays in smiling, social behaviour and visual tracking are encountered not only in babies with vision defects, but also in those with more generalized developmental backwardness and mental handicap.

Severe floppiness or **hypotonia** may be due to illness; mental handicap syndromes (central hypotonia) or disorders of peripheral nerve or muscle (neuromuscular causes). Of these by far the most common is **spinal muscular atrophy** of severe type—**Werdnig–Hoffman disease**. These babies present in infancy (sometimes with a quite acute onset) with floppiness of profound degree, but a bright alert appearance. Floppiness of sufficient degree to be detected on routine examination or noted by the parent is an indication for prompt referral.

Congenital dislocation of the hip (CDH)

Screening for CDH by clinical examination cannot detect all cases at birth however expert the examiner may be, and repeated observations are necessary. Awareness must be maintained until the child is seen to be walking normally. *Make sure parents understand this.*

The screening procedure

- The following are high risk groups and should be examined with particular care:
    - History of CDH in parent or sibling.
    - Breech delivery, particularly extended breech.
    - Congenital postural deformities of the feet or of other joints.
    - Other risk factors include oligohydramnios, fetal growth retardation and birth by Caesarean section.
    - In some districts, high-risk babies are examined by ultrasound. If this is the policy, it is important to ensure that it is carried out (*see* p. 194).
- Inspection for classical signs of dislocation; these are rarely detected at birth but become more common thereafter (p. 166).
- Examination to detect hip instability; **the modified Ortolani/Barlow manoeuvre**; this test should be used from birth up to the age of 3 months. It

is recommended that this should be performed within 24 hours of birth, again before the tenth day (though this is difficult to organize and the additional benefits are minimal) and at the 6–8-week examination. The tests must be performed gently, with warm hands and the baby relaxed (*see* Figure 6.2).

The procedure is described for examination of the left hip:

- The infant lies supine with the hips partially abducted and fully flexed, and the knees fully flexed.
- The examiner steadies the pelvis between the thumb of the left hand on the symphysis pubis and the fingers under the sacrum.
- The upper thigh of the left leg is grasped by the examiner's right hand with the middle finger over the greater trochanter, with the flexed leg held in the palm and with the thumb on the inner side of the thigh opposite the lesser trochanter.

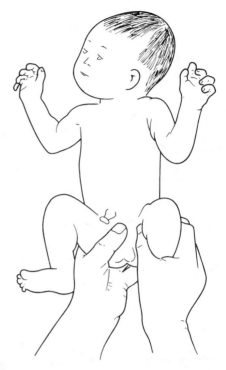

Figure 6.2. The modified Ortolani/Barlow manoeuvre.

The manoeuvre has two stages:

- **Ortolani test for dislocation**. The hip is gently abducted; simultaneously the middle finger presses on the greater trochanter in an attempt to relocate the head of the femur (which dislocates posteriorly) into the acetabulum. If dislocation is present the head will relocate with a movement of up to 5 mm and a definite clunk.
- **Barlow test for subluxable hip**. With the thumb on the inner side of the thigh, backward pressure is applied to the head of the femur. If the latter is felt to move backwards over the fibro-cartilaginous rim of the acetabulum, again with a movement of up to 5 mm and a clunk, the hip is subluxable or dislocatable. If this happens, the hip is gently abducted and will relocate. When the hip is adducted again, it will remain located.
- Ligamentous clicks without any movement of the head of the femur are of no significance.

If you do detect a case, do not encourage all your colleagues to come and manipulate the hip in and out of the acetabulum! Urgent referral to an orthopaedic surgeon is appropriate. Results are said to be better if treatment begins before 8 weeks.

A plastic model which demonstrates the feel of a dislocation and relocation is available: contact the Child Growth Foundation. It is expensive and should be purchased by the health authority or shared between several training practices.

N.B. All children with cerebral palsy and other severe disorders of the motor system should be considered at risk for dislocation of the hip **throughout childhood**.

Further reading

Dezateux C and Godward S (1998) Screening for congenital dislocation of the hip in newborn and young infants. In: TJ David (ed) *Recent Advances in Paediatrics, Volume 16*. Churchill Livingstone, Edinburgh.

Early diagnosis of congenital hearing loss

There are now several methods by which hearing loss can be detected in the first few weeks of life. Many districts now screen high-risk infants and it should be possible to detect between 30 and 60 per cent of all cases of congenital hearing loss by this approach. Universal neonatal screening is now thought to offer better value for money than the distraction test but will take some time to become established.

Neonatal screening

Some referrals are made from the Neonatal Intensive Care Unit and postnatal wards, and the remainder by the health visitors. At the first postnatal visit, the mother is given a leaflet which explains the concept of high-risk screening; on

---

Risk factors for hearing loss

- Infants requiring intensive care (not merely special care) for more than 48 hours, prematurity (gestation less than 33 weeks at birth or weight less than 1,500 g), severe asphyxia or respiratory depression at birth, meningitis, jaundice needing exchange transfusion, high levels of aminoglycosides.

- Family history of a hearing loss compatible with genetic transmission (i.e. include infants where the family history of a hearing loss is attributed to some other factor unless this is unequivocal—parents often falsely attribute the defect to measles, head injury, etc.).

- Chromosome defects and malformation syndromes; any infant with another major defect, particularly those which involve the head and face.

- Documented or suspected rubella, cytomegalovirus or other congenital infections in pregnancy.

- Consanguinity is associated with a small increase in risk.

the reverse of this leaflet is a check-list of infant behaviours (based on a check-list devised by McCormick)[1] which helps a parent to know that the baby has satisfactory hearing responses. The test is performed by a hearing screener, who uses one of the methods described on p. 62. Infants who fail the screening test must be referred promptly for full diagnostic evaluation.

Detection of serious vision defects

Ask the parents whether they have any concerns about the child's vision. Enquire about family history of vision defects and other high risk factors, in particular prematurity and other paediatric disorders.

Complaints suggestive of serious vision defect and needing immediate referral:

- Lack of fixation or following movements of the eyes.
- Wandering or roving eye movements.
- Abnormal appearance (white mass, cataracts, etc.).
- Nystagmus.
- Squint.
- Photophobia.
- Excessive watering of the eyes.
- Reluctance to open eyes.
- Lack of pigment in the eyes (appear pink in certain light).
- Abnormal reflection of light in a photograph taken with a flash.

Refer for expert examination the following babies:

- Premature infants (birth weight <1,250 g) who have required oxygen therapy, if they have not already been examined in the neonatal unit (cases of retinopathy of prematurity are still missed in units where there is not a strict policy).
- Infants with a positive family history for heritable eye disease.
- Children known to have other handicapping conditions.
- A permanent squint in one eye is never normal; prompt referral is necessary to exclude cataract and retinoblastoma.

Observe visual behaviour. Does the baby look at the parent's face and follow it as she moves from side to side in his field of vision?

Inspect the eyes carefully. (Ask the parent to hold the baby upright if he is reluctant to open his eyes—try not to force them open.) Are they the same size? If one eye is smaller than the other, it is likely to have poor vision. A slight asymmetry in the size of the pupils is normal.

Look for opacities, cloudiness of the cornea, defects in the iris. Note any photophobia. **Use the ophthalmoscope** set on plus 3, held at 10–12" to look for the red reflex, to exclude cataracts. This is not easy, especially in Afro-Caribbean babies whose retina is more heavily pigmented. Do not try to see the fundi; it is almost impossible to get an adequate look in the infant without dilating the pupils.

---

[1] Dr B McCormick, Children's Hearing Assessment Centre, General Hospital, Nottingham.

Health education topics

- **Immunization**: deal with any worries; sign up for course of primary immunizations.

- **Feeding and nutrition**: maintenance of breastfeeding, preparation of formula feeds.

- Parental **smoking** habits: exposure to cigarette smoke increases risk of child getting upper and lower respiratory tract infections and middle ear disease.

- Symptoms of **illness** in young babies.

- **Early infant development**.

- **Parents' needs**—sleep, return to work, etc.

- Problems with **siblings**.

- **Crying**—coping with frustration, tiredness.

- Reducing the risk of **cot death** (*see* p. 95).

- **Accident prevention:**

Danger	*Advice*
Fires	Smoke detectors; electrical safety.
Passenger injuries in road traffic accidents (RTA)	Safety restraints—cot harnesses; child safety seats and seat belts.
Falls	Do not leave unattended unless safely positioned. Small babies wriggle!
Scalds	Check temperature of bath and feeds carefully. Microwave ovens make fluids deceptively hot.
Drowning	*Never* leave unattended in a bath, even to answer the door or telephone.
Inhalation, ingestion and suffocation	Beware of small toys, furry toys, some dummies and long strings on dummies (the latter have been known to strangle babies).

8 weeks to 6 months

Contents

There are no routine examinations or health checks during this period but there are many incidental opportunities to examine babies, both during consultations for minor ailments and also when the baby attends for immunization. Problems which may present in this age group are more often related to general health or management issues than to developmental problems; for instance, colic, feeding difficulties, poor weight gain, constipation, crying at night, etc.

Normal development, 8 weeks–6 months

Learning and social development

In the first 6 months of life, the infant **learns** about daily rituals such as bathtime, feeding, changing, etc. He reveals this knowledge by showing **anticipation** when he see or hears the preparations for these events. He also enjoys games where anticipation is needed and he may begin to develop '**procedures**' to encourage their performance. For instance, he may rock back and forth with excitement or may vocalize loudly.

As early as 14 weeks, the baby may stare with obvious fascination at an unfamiliar person and by 6 months it is usually obvious even to the casual observer that he regards his familiar care-givers as different from other people. His laughter at his own reflection in a mirror suggests that he has some sense of himself as a person. However, at this stage he has not yet acquired a deep suspicion of strangers and it is usually quite easy to make friends with a baby of this age.

The formation of strong **attachments** is a natural part of the infant's development but these may be formed with either one or several people and indeed there may be advantages in a child having several attachment figures. The strength of attachment is related more to the quality of interaction between the baby and the care-giver, than to the actual amount of physical care. This point is important for parents who feel guilty about making use of a child-minder while they are at work.

Difficulties in managing or responding to the baby's needs may be a presenting symptom of maternal depression which may become more prominent when the baby is 3 or 4 months old (p. 129).

Motor development

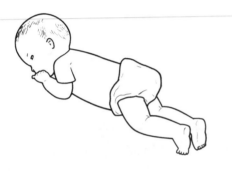

Age 3 months

- By 3 months the infant has developed a remarkable degree of voluntary control of his movements.
- Most of his waking time is spent moving arms and legs.
- He is able to maintain his head in a mid-position and is free to watch, follow and reach towards moving objects.
- He has more defined periods of wakefulness.

Supine

- Maintains head in mid-position.
- Moves head freely to watch dangling object, side to side and up and down.
- Stares at hands.
- Kicks legs into flexion and extension—mostly reciprocally, i.e. one leg up, one down as in cycling.

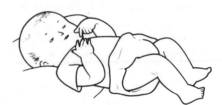

Prone

- Raises head to 60° and holds this position for minutes at a time.
- Weight is taken firmly on forearms.
- Pelvis rests flat on supporting surface.
- Hips extend and knees rotate outwards.
- Kicks with one or both legs, either reciprocally or symmetrically.

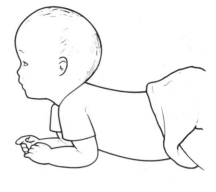

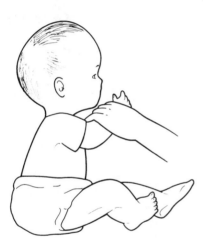

Sitting

- Placed in sitting position, balances head and has a little control of upper trunk.
- Head control is adequate to allow turning and following of a moving object.
- No balance of trunk.

Standing

- Takes some weight.
- Head remains balanced in line with trunk.
- No reflex stepping.

Grasp

- Grasps object if placed in hand.
- Uses total fisted grasp described as contact grasp. This grasp is partly involuntary.
- Will loose grasp (not release) after a few seconds.
- Unable to reach and grasp.
- Unable to move hand with object in it.

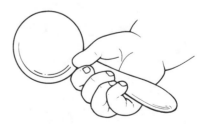

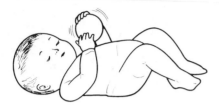

Age 4 months

- By 4 months symmetry is becoming established.
- The infant lies with head in mid-position and hands engaged in mid-line, typically with fingers in mouth.
- Legs flexed and abducted.

Supine

- Head mostly in mid-line.
- Hands engage in mid-line.
- Plays with fingers.
- Legs rest in flexed abducted posture.
- Kicks legs into full extension.
- Places feet on surface and hitches bottom for 1–2 seconds.
- May place one foot on opposite knee.
- May roll from back to side and side to back.
- Patterns of movement very varied, i.e. not stereotyped.

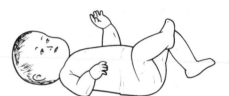

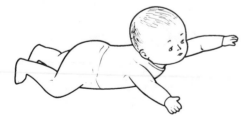

Prone

- Head firmly raised to 90°.
- Alternately takes weight firmly on elbows or extends arms and legs into aeroplane or swimming posture.
- Elbows starting to be placed forwards for weight bearing—no longer tucked under chest.
- Kicks legs in a variety of movement combinations using either or both legs.

Sitting

- Placed in sitting position supports head and trunk firmly.
- Lower back still needs support.
- Held firmly in sitting position he is able to control arm movements.
- May reach and touch toys placed just in front of his feet.
- May either collapse forwards or brace shoulders into retraction to gain stability.

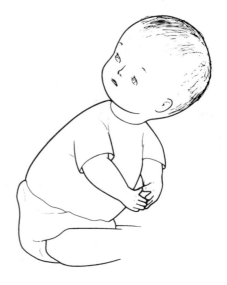

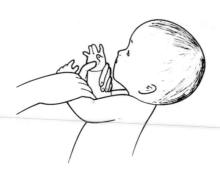

Standing

- Extends legs rhythmically and supports most of weight.
- Rises up onto toes.
- Grasps with toes.

Being moved

- Pulled up to the sitting position has only a slight head lag.
- Dangled on tummy (ventral suspension) shows intermittent extension of all limbs. Even when relaxed does not collapse into full flexion.
- When carried does not require support to head and shoulders.
- Makes small adjustments to changes of position on lap.

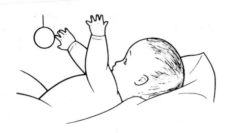

Grasp

- Primitive clutch.
- Starts to finger toys.
- Plucks at clothes and blankets.
- Plays with own hands.
- Grasps at attractive objects, may not hit the target!
- Takes all objects to mouth.
- Maintains rattle in hand for few minutes.

Age 5 months

- By 5 months the infant is physically very active.
- He spontaneously changes his position from lying flat on his stomach to pushing up onto extended arms.
- He reaches and grasps toys and has some ability to roll.

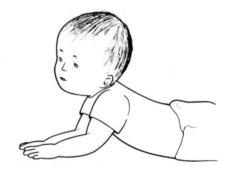

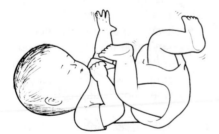

Supine

- Very active in this position.
- Grasps toys and brings them to mouth.
- Flexes legs and pelvis and plays with toes. Often places toes in mouth and sucks them.
- Places feet on mattress and lifts pelvis—bridging.
- Rolls from back to side with ease and almost to prone.
- May stay on side and play with toys or toes.

Prone

- Increasing variety of movement.
- Adopts aeroplane-position—arms and legs raised off floor and spread into abduction.
- Pushes up from forearms to extended arms.
- Transfers weight onto one arm and frees the other arm to reach for a toy.
- May start to move round in a circle—pivoting or pushing backwards on extended arms—pre-creeping.
- Rolls to supine.

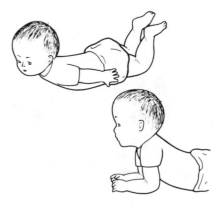

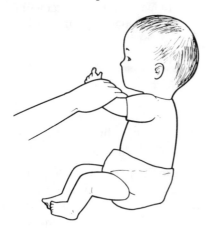

Sitting

- Needs only a little support to lower trunk.
- Head held firmly.
- Back held straight.
- Makes small adjustments to balance of trunk when tilted side to side.
- Early weight-bearing on hands to side—propping.

Being moved

- Pulled to the sitting position baby actively assists by bracing his shoulders and raising his head.
- Independent mobility is starting through rolling, pivoting and pre-creeping.

Standing

- Takes weight firmly.
- Makes pedalling movements with legs.

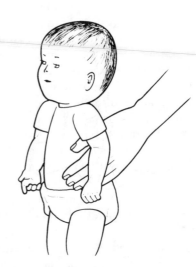

Grasp

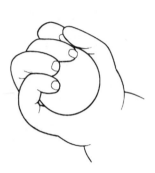

- Use of hands is best seen in supine or sitting with support. Hand function will otherwise be masked by the need to use hands to maintain balance.
- Reaches towards objects on table surface or dangled on a string.
- Grasps with palm and outer three fingers only, thumb and index finger not involved.
- Reaches, grasps and takes toy to mouth.
- Bangs toy.
- Release of toys is accidental and visual pursuit of a lost toy rare.

Clinical procedure

Clinical evaluation depends on the reason for the consultation, but the following observations take little time and help to reassure you and the parent.

- Observe the baby's **social behaviour in response to the parents** and to you or other strangers in the room. Vocalization, smiling and other facial expressions in response to the parent's voice should be more readily observed now than at 8 weeks. Vocalization at 3 months still consists of vowel sounds only, but the baby is beginning to gain some control over the voice and modulate the sounds as he coos in response to the parent.
- Ask about the baby's **response to sound**. At 4 months, he may orientate towards a sound, particularly when in the supine position. Parents often expect more rapid and precise localization than is realistic at this age, and this can result in unnecessary referrals to the audiology clinic.
- **Visual following** is now present through 180° and the baby can turn his head to follow an object at the extreme of lateral gaze.
- At around 3 months, the infant becomes **interested in his hands** and looks at them with intense interest. Place an object in the hand—it is grasped on contact but he cannot voluntarily release it. He is unlikely to reach for the object or to move it around but if it is held close to him but not near enough to grasp it, he may reveal by excited activity that the desire to obtain it is greater than the actual level of motor competence.
- When placed in the **sitting position**, the trunk and head control can be observed; safe independent sitting is unlikely to be achieved before 5 or 6 months, but the baby is progressing towards this goal.

Interpretation

Defects of vision and hearing may sometimes first be suspected by parents during this period.

Low muscle tone, lack of responsiveness, excessive stiffness and irritability, and being 'too good', can be early warning signs of developmental problems.

Colic

Colic is one of the most common problems in the first few months of life. Beware a complaint of 'colic' in which the baby flexes the **entire** trunk and may let out a cry; this may signify a sinister form of epilepsy—salaam attacks.

The cause of 3-month colic, which starts typically at about 3 weeks and persists as a daily problem until 14 weeks of age, is obscure, although clinical observation and the proven therapeutic effect of dicyclomine suggest that intestinal spasm is to blame. Intolerance to cows' milk has been implicated in a few cases but a considerable number of breast-fed babies are colicky. Wind from a teat with too large a hole in it is often blamed but altering the size of the hole has little or no effect. Undoubtedly the symptoms of gaseous distension of the stomach mimic colic, causing some distress, and are relieved by a burp but full-blown colic is not relieved by such simple measures.

Colic is not caused by anxious parents but it makes parents anxious, irritable and even desperate. Bad-tempered handling, rows between parents and shouting at the baby will exacerbate the baby's distress.

True colic with a screaming baby who cries and screams intensely for long periods, draws his knees right up and looks pale is to be differentiated from other causes of protracted crying and doubling up such as:

- Pain from an acute infection (ears, UTI, abdomen).
- The common phenomenon of a baby who becomes unsettled in the evening, continually rooting but not feeding fully who seems not to know whether he wants to be put down or picked up.
- Salaam attacks in infantile seizures which may result in the child appearing to draw up his knees during a jackknife spasm. There is only a brief cry.

Dicyclomine (Merbentyl) is now contraindicated in babies under 6 months because of a possible link with some cases of respiratory and neurological collapse.

The encouraging finding in the studies which established dicyclomine as superior to placebo is the size of the placebo effect. Doing almost nothing may help a bit but there is no definite cure for the full clinical problem.

The following steps are sensible:

- Examine the baby, asking the parents what they fear might be wrong.
- Explain that the problem is colic which is common, caused by spasm in the gut, and short-lived.
- Emphasize that it is not caused by poor feeding or handling; make sure this message gets through to the father.
- Say that there is no known definite cure but that it will pass by 14 weeks (16 to be absolutely sure).

- Consider offering to put all this in a letter to them so that they can show it to in-laws and neighbours.
- Remind them that **it is a parent's first duty to survive** and they should:
  - Take turns in attempting to soothe the baby, out of earshot of the other if possible, by rhythmic rocking, massaging the tummy, giving gripe-water, rides in the pram, etc. A small baby can be carried prone over and along a horizontal forearm and have his back rubbed while being carried around.
  - Put a calendar on the wall with the 14-week deadline marked, and cross off each day as it passes.
  - Ensure that the mother gets some sleep during the day so that she is not exhausted by the evening. She can sleep while her baby sleeps.
- Offer follow-up by yourself or the health visitor within a week or two.

Health education topics

- Accident prevention.

Parents should be thinking about the next stage in development—the child will soon be mobile.

Danger	*Advice*
Falls	Do not leave unattended in baby walker. Block access to stairs.
Scalds/burns	Do not leave hot food or drinks within reach. Guard all fires and radiators.
Inhalation, ingestion and suffocation	Keep small objects (peanuts, pen tops, small toys, etc.) out of reach.
Overheating	Warn parents about dangers: heaters left on by mistake in warm weather; baby left to sleep in car during summer months.

- Reinforce the advice given previously (p. 140).
- Discuss infant feeding practice and sugar intake.
- Recommend registration with a dentist.

---

6 to 12 months

This section reviews the normal developmental progress of the infant between 6 and 12 months of age. The importance of attachment behaviour is stressed. The review at 6–9 months is described and detailed instructions are given for the performance of the distraction test of hearing and for the recheck of the hips. Health education topics are summarized.

Normal development, 6–12 months

Learning and communication

The baby's understanding and use of **speech sounds** continue to mature. He listens carefully to speech and his own vocalizations now include a variety of sounds, usually with a few consonants such as B, D or M. The range and quality of these sounds is diminished in the deaf infant.

The ability to **localize the source of sound** also improves so that by 7–9 months he can locate sounds to either side and behind him quite accurately, though he may still have difficulty localizing sounds made directly above or below him. The 'auditory world' also expands and the infant becomes aware of sound stimuli at an increasing distance from him.

The maturation of localization is clinically important, because infants with slow development may be unable to locate a sound during the standard screening test of hearing. A failed hearing test may therefore sometimes be the presenting feature of general backwardness or mental handicap rather than deafness.

Visual behaviour

Visual acuity has probably not reached adult levels by 9 months, but depth perception and a sense of parallax are established. The visual world expands, so that the baby now shows an ability to look at and follow objects or people some distance away, for instance on the far side of a room. Objects in the far distance are less likely to attract visual attention at this stage.

Very tiny objects can capture the baby's attention, for example tiny bits of fluff on a carpet, or biscuit crumbs. As with hearing, a reduced visual awareness of small objects and apparent lack of interest in visual stimuli at a distance of more than a few feet, may be a sign of general slowness in development rather than of a vision defect.

Parents make use of the increasing visual alertness in promoting language development. As the infant's gaze falls on an object or person, the parent names it and talks about it. In this way, the relationship between the object and its word label gradually becomes established. This phenomenon is called **referential looking** (Figure 8.1).

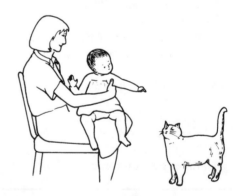

Figure 8.1. Referential looking. The child looks at the cat, the mother follows his line of gaze and says, 'Yes, that's a cat'.

Object permanence

Between 6 and 9 months, the baby discovers an important principle—that objects have a continued existence of their own, even when out of sight. This concept is known as object permanence.

By 7 months, the baby will search briefly for an object which has been dropped. By 9 months he will make a more determined and prolonged search. At first, covering an object seems to make it disappear from the infant's awareness; by 9 or

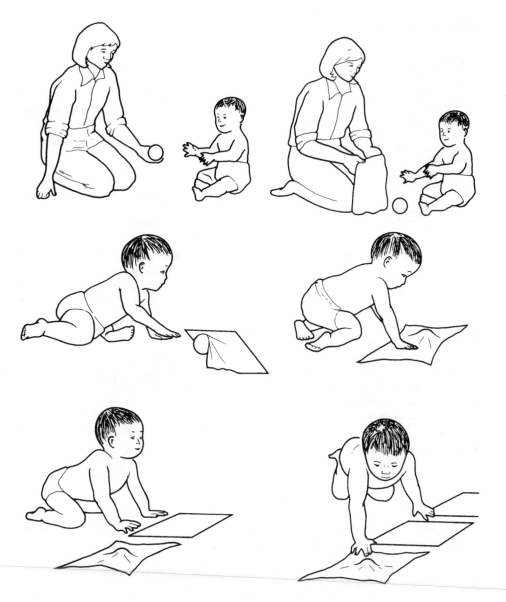

Figure 8.2. Stages in the development of 'object permanence'.

Motor development

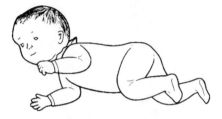

Age 6–7 months

- By 6 months the baby is developing the ability to initiate changes of position and make his desires clear-ly known in respect of whether he will sit up, lie down, etc.
- He is no longer happy to stay in one position and rolls from prone to supine and back again.
- He is starting to move in the horizontal plane in several directions and may even pursue a discarded toy.

Supine

- Does not stay in this posi-tion for long—rolls to prone.
- Raises head from floor in an invitation to be sat up!
- Pulls up on adult's fingers to sitting position.
- Plays with fingers and toes.
- Still places foot on opposite knee.

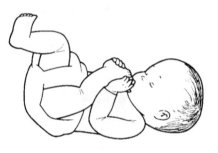

10 months however, and certainly by the end of the first year, the infant should quickly be able to locate an object covered by a cloth (Figure 8.2).

The task can be made more complex as the baby gets older. For instance, he can be confused deliberately by hiding the object under one of several cloths. By 15 months, the well-developed sense of object permanence is shown by the child's ability to locate lost toys and to know where prized possessions are kept.

Object permanence develops in parallel with **person permanence**. The baby begins to realize that his parent exists, even when not in the same room. The establishment of a mental image of familiar people is a necessary prerequisite of eventual separation and independence from the parent.

Play

Other areas of learning can be observed by watching the baby play. He experiments with the effects of pulling, shaking and dropping objects; he dis-covers the mechanism of cause and effect; he examines the size, shape and weight of objects and their relationship to each other. By 1 year of age he can concentrate for surprisingly long periods on a single task.

Prone
- Active!
- Pushes up onto arms.
- Moves round in circles.
- Pushes backwards.
- Starting to heave self forwards either using both arms together or alternate arms.
- Legs may only assist minimally at this stage.

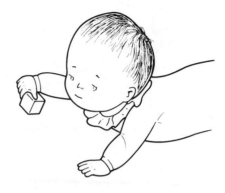

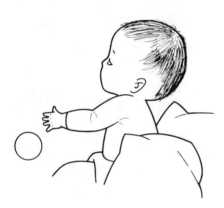

Sitting
- Sits without support for increasing periods.
- Needs cushions around him to protect from heavy falls to sides or backwards.
- Has good control forwards.

Standing
- Bounces on feet.
- Flexible.
- Rarely takes all of weight.

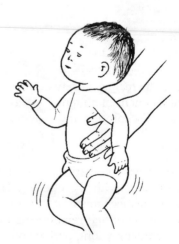

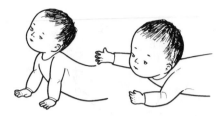

Grasp
- Grasp remains crude, described as a palmar or scoop grasp.
- The functional area of the hand is moving across and the thumb is minimally involved.
- Considerable variation of manipulation.
- Picks up objects of differing sizes, shapes and weights.
- Transfers objects hand to hand and hand to mouth.
- Manipulates with either hand or both together.
- Can modify grasp effort from banging a toy hard on the table to gentle flicking of a rattle or patting a mirror.

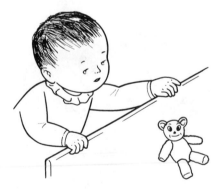

Moving
- Starting to move alone flat on belly using 'commando' creeping or pivoting.

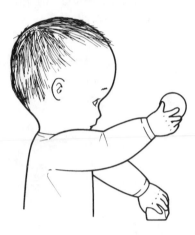

Age 8–9 months

By 8 months the baby has increasing fluency between movements.

- He can move between positions, e.g. sitting to crawling to sitting, and change from the horizontal, lying, to the upright, sitting.
- Attention span is increasing and individual objects are investigated for long periods.
- The baby has started to gain control of movement of his own body in his environment and control of objects that he encounters.

Supine
- Does not like this position—feels stranded and vulnerable.
- Either sits up or rolls over to escape from supine.

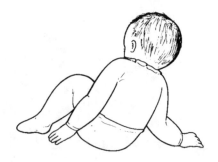

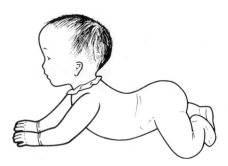

Prone/moving
- Freely adopts this position from supine or sitting.
- May continue to creep, or have developed an all-fours position, i.e. prone kneeling.
- May rock on all fours or start to crawl—backwards initially.
- Moves between sitting and crawling and crawling and sitting.
- Moves around in sitting, twisting and shuffling to pursue a toy.
- Some babies develop this ability to move in sitting position to a greater degree and become 'bottom shufflers' (p. 194).

Sitting
- Sits for longer periods from 1 minute upwards, can get into and out of this position.
- Saving and propping on hands well developed forwards and emerges sideways by around 9 months.
- Sitting no longer a static position but a dynamic posture.

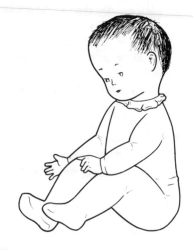

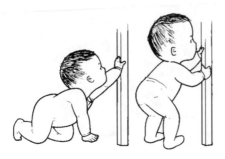

Standing
- Pulls up to standing on furniture, in cot as well as on adults.
- Leans trunk against support and takes weight firmly on soles of feet.
- Toes may claw intermittently especially on effort, e.g. rising to standing.
- Toes intermittently relax and wriggle.
- Weight is no longer taken symmetrically at all times and is shifted slightly from one leg to the other.
- Rises to standing with ease but has great difficulty in getting down.

Grasp
- Pincer grasp emerging.
- Thumb touches side of index finger.
- Grasp has shifted from the outer side of the hand across to the inner.
- The index finger is active in poking and prodding toys.
- Release of objects is starting. May still need a little nudge on the floor or from an adult's hand to complete release.
- Baby tosses toys for a short distance and then retrieves them.
- He watches the effect intently and pursues them even when they go out of sight.

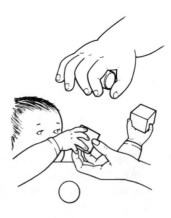

Reflex reactions
- Balance reactions developing in sitting.
- Saving reactions developing forwards and sideways in sitting.

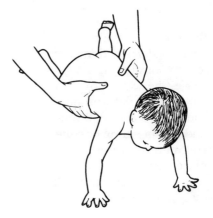

Downward parachute reaction

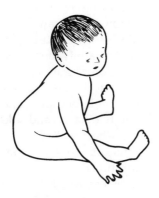

Forwards reaction

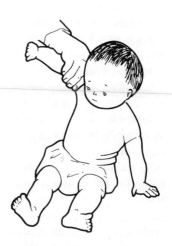

Sideways reaction

Age 10–11 months

- By 10 months the baby has developed a new dimension to his control of his body in space—he can move fluently from flat (prone or supine) to standing through kneeling or sitting or either.
- He can travel from place to place either by crawling, cruising or more unusually by bottom shuffling.

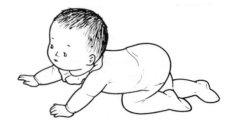

Supine
- More tolerant of this position but still rarely stays in it.

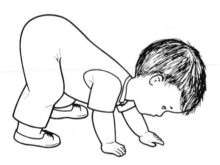

Prone/moving
- Increasing variations of creeping and crawling.
- Moves forwards using any or all of a variety of methods—four-point crawling using alternate hands and knees; two hands, one knee and one foot; two hands and soles of feet—'bear walking'.
- Pulls up to standing on furniture.
- Transfers weight from foot to foot.

- By 11 months moves sideways along furniture or cot—'cruises'.
- Still uses three points of balance: two feet and chest; two feet and one arm; two hands and one foot.
- Gradually over these 2 months these points of balance move more distally, i.e. away from leaning on a chair or low table with trunk to standing well back from the table using only hands or finger tips for support.
- Starting to drop from standing to sitting with control.
- Pushes stable wheeled toys, e.g. brick truck.
- Walks with adult if two hands held.

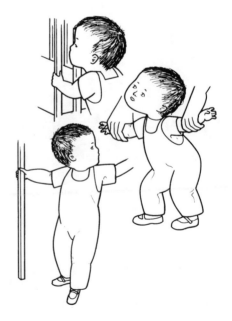

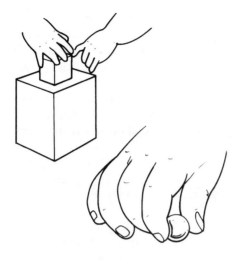

Grasp
- Places objects into and out of container.
- Release of objects becoming more controlled.
- Teases adult by offering toy but not releasing.
- Alternately drops object for adult to retrieve!
- Pincer grasp emerging involving thumb and tip of index finger.
- Uses index finger to point and poke.
- Grasp now more economical—only opens fingers enough for the task in hand.
- Starting to estimate size and weight of objects.

Reflex reactions
- Balance reactions emerging in standing.
- Saving reactions in sitting well developed forwards, sideways and emerging backwards.
- Saving reactions in standing becoming more effective.

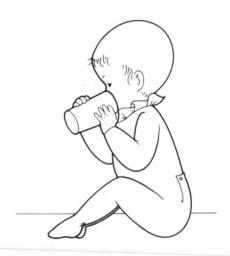

Attachment and affectional bonding

Attachment theory states that the clinging behaviour which young children display towards their parents is normal and biologically determined, has particular characteristics, and is especially important in psychosocial development. Selective clinging to one person is understood as evidence of an individual's first close personal relationship and it is held that the experience of that relationship will govern the quality of subsequent close relationships throughout life.

Attachment behaviour refers to what you actually see: the clinging, or conversely, the **separation anxiety** shown by the child at separation from his or her **attachment figure**.

Small babies accept separation from parents with apparent equanimity. At an average age of about 6–7 months they start to show signs (i.e. attachment behaviours) which indicate that they are becoming psychologically attached to another person, usually their mother. In most cases it is one particular individual (occasionally two, simultaneously) in the first instance.

This person is singled out from others by the baby as being especially significant and important. She or he does not have to be related by blood and certainly does not have to be the biological mother. There is little or no relationship with events during the neonatal period. The attachment figure is usually someone who has had a lot to do with the baby in terms of play and comforting; feeding is not the crucial element and breast or bottle-feeding is simply irrelevant. Even harsh physical treatment or battering is compatible with the development of an attachment to the abuser; so long as the carer has involved themselves in intense social interactions with the infant, that may be sufficient. Nor is the amount of time spent with a person crucial, what matters is the intensity of social interactions. Working mothers are quite able to elicit attachments from their infants so long as they do things with them at some time during the average day. In practice, the first attachment figure is nearly always the baby's mother (or attachment is formed equally with mother and father) and for the sake of simplicity the term mother is used here. After the first attachment a few other attachments are likely to be formed, particularly to the other parent, but usually do not have the intensity of the first one.

Normal attachment behaviours comprise:

- Crying when mother leaves the room; calling for her.
- Crawling or toddling after her.
- Clinging hard when anxious, fearful, tired or in pain.
- Hugging, climbing onto her lap talking and playing more in her company.
- Using her as a secure base from which to explore.

All are intensified by anxiety, tiredness and illness.

These are evidence of normal psychosocial development in toddlers between about 6 months and 3 years, and are quite compatible with secure attachment formation and can be detected during medical consultations. They may be less obviously selective when the baby or small child has been reared in a larger or extended family. They abate gradually after the age of about 3.

At the same time in development as the appearance of attachment behaviour (average 6 months), there is usually the development of **stranger anxiety**, a wariness towards and shyness of strange people which promotes clinging to the attachment figure in their presence. This can also be noted during ordinary medical consultations and is likewise a normal developmental feature, quite compatible with the formation of a secure attachment.

The mother's presence calms the child; her absence (or threatened absence) precipitates separation anxiety. This is normal but can interfere with settling at night. Some children find that they can deal with it by having a cuddly toy, known as a **comfort object** or **transitional object**, such as a blanket or teddy bear. These are useful devices and do not usually need to be discouraged, even though parents sometimes disapprove of them. **Their existence does not indicate insecurity.**

Usually, a child gradually learns to tolerate separations, so that separation anxiety wanes over the preschool years, although it will still appear at times of distress and pain in young schoolchildren. The rate at which this happens depends on three variables:

- The temperament (personality) of the child.
- The way in which the mother handles the child.
- What experiences the child has of actual or threatened separations.

Adequate resolution of separation anxiety is promoted by the mother being **sensitively responsive** to the child's needs and providing a sense of **security**. It follows that if a mother responds to clinging by pushing the child away brusquely, if she uses threats of abandonment as coercions, or if her health and constancy are threatened in the child's eyes, then the child continues to feel **insecure** and anxious.

The resolution of separation anxiety and observable attachment behaviour goes hand in hand with the development of faith that the mother will always return after separation; in other words, a relationship has developed which can persist in the temporary absence of the mother. It is usually thought that this depends upon the child having formed an internal mental representation of his other; an idea and an image. The term **bonding** was originally used to describe this process and it was held that the development by the child of **affectional bonds** allowed the proximity-seeking attachment behaviour to subside. Unfortunately, the term 'bonding' has more recently also been used to describe the warm feelings a mother may have towards her newborn baby—a different, less significant, and probably unrelated process (*see* p. 115).

The development of secure affectional bonds in early childhood makes it much more likely that an attitude of trust and optimism in personal relationships will persist in later life. Conversely, a failure to develop affectional bonds may result in a lack of what is often called **basic trust** with resulting shallowness, suspicion and selfishness in future relationships.

Although the acquisition of affectional bonds means that the child no longer has to maintain proximity to his or her mother, if she dies or otherwise disappears, **grief** ensues.

Although most children form one initial attachment, others follow. The usual sequence is for mother to be the first, father to follow some months later, and then figures such as grandparents or siblings. It is often assumed that each successive attachment is rather weaker than the previous one. Nevertheless, some children form two or more attachments simultaneously, especially in families where child care is shared between a number of adults. In such families, separation anxiety is less evident because the departure of the child's mother merely means that the care of the child is likely to be in the hands of another attachment figure. The child still feels secure even though the person changes.

The process of attachment formation and the establishment of affectional bonds usually takes place over the years between age 6 months and 4 years. After that time it is more difficult to form deep attachments and bonds to parental figures, though not impossible; many late adoptions are successful from that point of view. The whole process is echoed in late adolescence and adult life by falling in love which is sometimes called **pair bonding**. In turn, this is followed by the development of deep affection for one's own children.

Abnormalities of attachment formation

Absent or attenuated attachments

Attachment behaviours may fail to develop adequately. The child may appear endearingly friendly to the examining doctor but closer questioning or longer acquaintance reveals that he or she does not discriminate between familiar and unfamiliar adults in terms of seeking comfort and affection. Although appearing intimate (sitting on your lap, offering kisses) the relationship is superficial and easily broken by separation without any separation anxiety. There are two main reasons for this:

- unsuitable circumstances: institutional rearing (especially in the case of late adoptions); emotionally cold or rejecting parents;
- abnormal child: profound mental handicap; autism.

In either case, referral to a child psychiatrist is sensible. In the instance of unsuitable circumstances, the long-term outcome is often poor with a general difficulty forming and sustaining close relationships, a difficulty learning social rules and a propensity in adult life to aggressive, promiscuous, or feckless behaviour. This is essentially what used to be called **maternal deprivation**. It may be associated with other consequences of poor parental care.

Avoidant attachment

There is no indiscriminate attachment behaviour; the child has formed a selective attachment. Clinging and separation anxiety are muted, the child separating from his mother reasonably easily and playing by himself in her absence. On her return he is indifferent to her presence or even actively avoids her greeting. On other occasions he is likely to behave aggressively towards her, although not all the time. The clinical task is differentiating between avoidant attachment from what can look like secure self-sufficient behaviour. Simply asking the mother whether she feels emotionally close to her child is the easiest test. Secure children have gone through a phase of clinging and subsequently share emotions and experiences readily with their mother without demanding reassurance or excessive attention. Avoidant children have always kept their mothers at a distance and seem to strive for emotional self-sufficiency prematurely.

In some instances this pattern reflects elements in the *child's* personality; he dislikes cuddles and intimacies even though the parents are loving and affectionate. He wriggles off laps and dislikes kisses. Such a pattern has a good prognosis so long as the parents can accept their child's individuality. There is no strong link with aggressive behaviour.

In other instances the pattern arises on account of harshness, coldness or rejection on the part of the *parent*. This is evident when mother and child are seen together and it is this configuration which is associated with a tendency for the child to behave aggressively to his mother in other settings. This has a poor prognosis for future antisocial behaviour. The situation can be improved if the parent can be persuaded to act in a more sensitive, affectionate and child-centred way but this is not easy. In theory, professional counselling is indicated but such parents will not readily accept it and continue to berate their child.

Insecure attachment

The child is chronically clingy and obviously ambivalent to the mother, being actively cross with her following the briefest separations. The origins of this usually lie in an unfortunate mix of the child's temperament and mother's state of mind or personality. A depressed and irritable mother, for instance, may be short-tempered with a querulous child and her rejecting attitude promotes further cling-ing by the child. A mother with an immature personality may find herself unable to separate out her needs from the child's and turns to the child for caring or gratification in a way that makes the child anxious and clingy. Some insecure infants, however, have been exceptionally anxious and irritable throughout their lives and have perfectly satisfactory mothers; it is wrong to *always* blame the child's mother for causing an insecure attachment.

It has generally been held that insecure attachments are likely to precede emotional disorder in childhood, particularly school refusal. Some believe that disorders arising in adolescence or adult life such as agoraphobia also have their roots in insecure attachment formation in early childhood. For such reasons it is appropriate to refer insecure children to a child psychiatrist if the problem has not resolved by the age of 5.

A sensitive period?

There seems to be a relatively sensitive period for the effects of poor quality rearing of the type which does not allow for the development of adequate attach-ments. For instance, an institutional upbringing during the first few months of life only, or admission to an institution in middle childhood after an adequate home life in the early years are not associated with the above problems. As a rough guide it would appear that the years between ages 1 and 4 are the crucial ones, although there is wide variation and many adoptions later than age 4 can work well.

Summary of examination between 6 and 9 months

- Review with parent(s):
  - Their family life.
  - The baby's health, growth and progress.
- Follow up any expressed concerns.
- Observe:
  - Socialization and attachment behaviour.
  - Visual behaviour.
  - Communication—sounds, expressions and gestures.
  - Motor development—sitting, balance, hand functions, any abnormal movement patterns.
- Check for risk factors for hearing and vision defects.
- Look at eyes and eye movements.
- Check the hips.
- Distraction test of hearing.

- Physical examination to include heart and testes.
- Complete physical examination, length, weight and head circumference, if indicated.
- Health education topics.

Review between 6 and 9 months

Every baby should be seen between 6 and 9 months. This is an age when most babies are learning to sit and to communicate. In addition, it is the optimal age for hearing tests by the distraction method. The focus of the review is development and growth, and these lead naturally to a discussion of the next stages of development and the implications for learning and for accident prevention. The physical checks may be carried out at any convenient time in this age-band, on an opportunistic basis.

- A **complete physical examination** is indicated *if* some problem has been raised by the parents or has been suggested by an appraisal of the child's health or developmental progress.
- The following elements of physical examination should be performed in every case whether or not there are complaints or worries:
  - Check for descent of testes; if doubt remains after 6 week check.
  - Look for signs of congenital dislocation of the hip.
  - Auscultate the heart, and check for signs of congenital heart disease (*see* p. 135).

These physical checks will usually be done by the GP, either in a special child health session or on an opportunistic basis when the baby is seen for some other reason; *ensure* that the findings are recorded. There is no reason why the health visitor should not learn to check the hips and testes.

Hips

Inspection for **classical signs of dislocation;** these are rarely present at birth but become more common thereafter. They are much easier to detect when unilateral because of the resulting asymmetry. The signs described here are not always present, are difficult to elicit and can be missed even by expert examiners.

Signs of hip dislocation

- The thigh on the abnormal side lies in partial lateral rotation, flexion and abduction.
- Above-knee shortening is seen by comparing the level of the knees with the hip flexed.
- There may be asymmetry of the thigh and groin creases, although on its own this is not a very reliable sign.
- The buttock on the affected side may appear flattened when the baby is prone.
- Reduced range of abduction is detected by placing the infant on his back with the hips flexed to 90° and gently abducting the thighs simultaneously. The

range of normal is wide but the average is 75°. Abduction may also be reduced in irritable hypertonic babies.

- The resistance to abduction may give way with a clunk as the head of the femur relocates. This sign becomes less common as the infant gets older but may persist until the second year.
- With bilateral dislocation there may be a perineal gap between the thighs.

Review of developmental progress

- **Review the baby's development** with his parents. The parents now have an extensive store of knowledge about their baby's temperament, behaviour and development and this information helps you to evaluate the child's development quickly and accurately. Many parents have already begun to suspect defects such as hearing loss or squint, or are concerned about delay in motor development.
- It is usually best to **talk about the baby's health and growth**, together with any management problems first, thus allowing the baby a few minutes to settle and become used to the presence of a stranger. He should be seated on the floor or on his parent's lap, with a few simple toys within reach.
- Ask **open questions** first. Are there any worries about growth, health, appetite or development? How are the parents coping and how do they feel? Are there any family or sibling difficulties?
- **Watch** the baby's response to you and to his parents. Suspicion and wariness are normal at this age. Take your time; do not alarm the baby by making friendly advances too soon. Move slowly, speak gently and retreat if he becomes restive and anxious. Offer a small toy, as a gesture of friendly intent.
- While establishing rapport with the baby, **ask the parents** about this ability to distinguish between them and familiar adults such as grandparents. At this age most babies know their familiar family figures and respond differently to them as compared with strangers.
- As many babies are unusually quiet in unfamiliar surroundings, ask about **vocalizations**. Does he modulate his cooing sounds (eee-ahah), chatter with consonant sounds, for example ba, ma, or da? (these appear around 7 to 10 months). From 6 to 7 months most babies enjoy sound games: they copy raspberry noises or imitate a cough.
- Does he begin to **understand** voice (not the actual meaning of words)? Ask the parents to call him and observe the response. Does he listen when they talk to him and does he try to have a conversation?
- Enquire also about his other methods of **communication**. Does he convey his excitement at mealtimes or bathtime? Does he insist on attention by shouting or indicate by other means that he wants a particular object? Can he play anticipation games such as 'peep-bo'?
- Ask the parents to offer him a favourite toy. Observe the use of his **hands**—is he accurate in reaching and grasping; does he use both hands equally well? It is not normal for a baby to be obviously left- or right-handed at this age. The grasp becomes increasingly direct and accurate between 6 and 9 months.
- At 6 months, all toys tend to be handled in much the same way, with little discrimination between them at this age. Each object is taken to the mouth.

By 9 months there may be some differential response to different kinds of toys.

- The index finger may be used preferentially by 7 or 8 months in an attempt to poke at a sweet and by 9 months most babies can pick up a sweet between thumb and first finger, though the grasp is not yet mature.
- Look next at gross **motor development**.
- You will already have observed whether he has **sitting balance** while he is sitting on the parent's lap. The mother can tell you immediately whether she can leave him on the floor unsupported.
- If he does not sit well without support, try taking him on your lap and sitting him for a moment. Feel whether he has trunk balancing movements as you adjust his position; tilt him slightly and notice his head control. **Sit him on the floor or couch** and gently tilt him again from side to side. He should extend the arm on each side as a propping reaction to stabilize himself. If an object is placed behind or to one side he should be able to recover it without falling.

   (There is, of course, a wide variation in the rate of motor development; it would not be unusual for a baby to be rather unstable in sitting at 7 or 8 months but the absence of any sitting balance, saving reaction or trunk righting would be worrying.)

- In the **prone position** he should be able to roll over; ask the parent if he can do this. By 8 months many babies can push up on the arms sufficiently to lift the pelvis clear of the floor in readiness for crawling. While in the prone position, check the **forwards saving (parachute)** response (*see* diagram on p. 159). This is usually easily demonstrated beyond about 8 months and is useful evidence that there is no asymmetry between the right and left arms.
- From lying on the floor or couch, he can be **pulled to sitting** with no more than a little finger support for traction and may manage to achieve sitting from lying without any assistance at all.
- Hold the baby in **vertical suspension** and lower him suddenly to the floor. Babies who are following the usual course of development, of crawling then standing, brace their legs with the feet plantigrade as they approach the surface. Babies who are shufflers (p. 194) bring their legs to the horizontal position as if sitting on air.
- Check the **hips**. Measure the **length** and **head circumference** if indicated.

Interpretation

Developmental examination at 6 to 9 months is very dependent on the infant's ability to give **motor** responses to stimuli. It may therefore be difficult to decide if an infant who is late in achieving motor milestones has a purely movement problem or whether this is simply a reflection of more general backwardness. Conversely, gross motor development may be normal or even advanced in spite of quite severe intellectual backwardness.

The two most commonly encountered developmental abnormalities at this age are:

- **Delay in reaching gross motor milestones**. There is no precise age at which one can say that delay in reaching a milestone such as sitting is pathological.

As a rough guide, most babies can sit by 10 months, and almost all by 12 months; stand by 13–14 months; walk by 18 months.

Generalized or global retardation (mental handicap, mental backwardness) is an important cause of delayed gross motor development. There are likely to be corresponding deficits in fine motor skills and social behaviour. Responses to hearing and vision assessment may also be poor or immature (p. 174). Muscle tone is usually normal or reduced but profound floppiness is rare and there is usually a good range of spontaneous movement. Babies who present in this way may have a non-progressive mental handicap syndrome.

Cerebral palsy can usually be diagnosed by the age of 9 months. There is delay in motor milestones; a reduced range, speed and accuracy of movement, particularly of the hands; the muscle tone can be increased or decreased and often varies with position and handling. The baby does not *feel* right and his movements do not *look* right. Do not be misled by the absence of an abnormal birth history. Less than 10 per cent of cerebral palsy cases are attributable to perinatal asphyxia.

- **Asymmetry of motor function**. This is usually first observed in the hand rather than the leg. Failure to use a hand, or apparent strong hand preference in the first year, is sufficient indication for referral. The baby may have congenital spastic hemiplegia or a brachial plexus lesion (Erb's palsy). There is also a benign developmental asymmetry called 'preferred head turning'. These babies always turn more to one side, have a strong hand preference and walk 'crabwise'.

Hearing assessment

Ask the parent these questions:

- Do you have any worries at all about your child's hearing?
- Why are you sure that your child *can* hear? (Some examples are given in the box below.)

Questions about hearing

What do *you* think about his hearing?
Why do you think he can/cannot hear?

- e.g. listens and turns to voices.
- Wakes when bedroom door opens.
- Hears dog bark, parent's key in lock, etc.
- Hears rustling of sweet or biscuit paper.
- Responds to name.

Can he tell where a sound is coming from?
Does he respond better if you raise your voice?
Does his hearing seem to vary from day to day?

Consider if there are any high risk factors for **sensorineural deafness** in the past or family history.

The risk factors listed below are indications for referral to the audiology clinic at *any* age if neonatal testing has not been done.

Are there any pointers in the history that suggest an increased risk of **secretory otitis media** (otitis with effusion, glue ear)?

Risk factors for secretory otitis media

- Repeated ear infections with or without earache, constant nasal discharge, mouth breathing and difficulty with eating, together with snoring at night even when the child does not have a cold.
- Episodes of sleep apnoea lasting for 10–15 seconds followed by partial waking. These are associated with severe persistent airway obstruction and a high risk of middle ear disorder.
- A complaint of discharge from the ear may occasionally be a sign of chronic suppurative middle ear disease but a brown discharge without any odour usually consists only of soft wax. (Many parents feel that the comment that the child has wax in the ear implies an accusation of poor hygiene!)
- Cleft palate, craniofacial anomalies; Down's, Turner's and Williams' syndromes.

Distraction test

All babies should have a hearing test in the first year of life. Within the next few years this will probably be accomplished by universal neonatal screening. The distraction test is the best option until then, but it is expensive in professional time if done well; the yield is low; there are many false positives; it is very difficult for staff to maintain standards of testing and vigilance when true positive cases are so rarely found.

Principles

The test relies on the ability of the child to turn and locate a sound made outside the field of vision. When used as a screening procedure, the distraction test should be carried out at between 6 and 10 months. There are good developmental reasons for this advice.

Babies of less than 6 months will often show a change in behavioural pattern when they hear an interesting sound but this response is too unpredictable for use in screening and would be interpreted with considerable caution even in an audiology clinic.

By 6 or 7 months, the baby has learnt to sit and has acquired control of trunk and head posture. By 8 months of age, 95 per cent of babies have acquired the ability to localize a sound source accurately, in any position except directly behind or above the head. At this age, it is possible to repeat the sound stimulus a number of times, because the baby does not retain a mental image of the tester or the sound maker which are outside his field of vision. He will therefore respond on each occasion as if to a novel stimulus.

By 10 or 12 months the concepts of object and person permanence are established, so that the baby can retain a memory of the tester's activities behind him; after the first few sounds have been made he begins to search for the sound maker before the stimulus is presented, or alternatively he quickly learns to ignore the sound unless a wider range of stimuli are used to maintain novelty. This increasing developmental sophistication makes the whole procedure longer and there is more scope for misinterpretation. By this age also deaf babies have learned to make 'check turns' to see what is happening around them.

Conditions

- Two people are *essential*. One makes the sounds—the **tester**. The other controls the baby's attention and makes the decisions about whether responses are significant—the **distractor** or observer. This person should be the more experienced of the two.

  There is no place for screening tests performed without a distractor nor for reliance on any handy receptionist or cleaner as an assistant. If this is the best that can be provided it is better not to run a screening programme at all.
- Staff must have their own hearing checked every two years.
- Staff must be adequately trained. Both testers should be familiar with the use of the sound-level meter.
- The room must be the quietest available, and use the quietest time during the week when no other activities are going on. Aim for a relaxed non-clinical atmosphere. The light source should be behind the distractor to avoid shadows. Watch out for vibrations, creaking floorboards, rustling clothes, jewellery, reflections, visual clues given by siblings, powerful perfume or after-shave, unconscious assistance given by parent.
- The baby should be alert, well, and have adequate head control.
- Explain the purpose and design of the test to the parent. By creating a partnership with the parent, you secure their cooperation and they are less likely to reject the result.

The test

The aim is to check and cross-check the frequencies important for speech. Test each ear for high and low frequency sounds separately, avoiding any fixed rhythm of presentation.

It is possible for an experienced tester to detect unilateral hearing loss, by observing a tendency always to locate sounds to one side; but the main objective of the screening test is to detect children with bilateral loss, which of course is far more likely to impair language acquisition.

Place all equipment conveniently behind you before starting.

The baby is placed on the parent's lap facing the distractor across a low table, supported round the waist but held well away from the parent (*see* Figure 8.3).

The **distractor** holds the baby's attention with a gently moving toy. When his attention is riveted on the toy, the distractor reduces the stimulation by covering or removing the toy, but does not let the child handle it. The fingers covering the toy should be gently moved to hold the baby's gaze on the hands, rather than the face; once the baby makes eye contact, he may be too interested in the distractor to turn towards the sound.

The **tester** presents sound stimuli at a distance of 3 feet from the child's ear, i.e. at arm's length from the edge of the parent's chair, on the same horizontal plane, at a sufficient angle that the child cannot see but not so far behind as to confuse

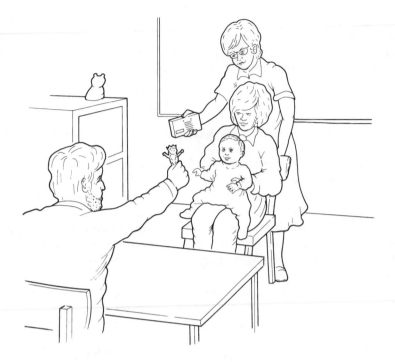

Figure 8.3. The distraction test, remembering to capture the child's attention before the sound stimulus is made.

the child's ability to locate (babies have difficulty in locating a sound source directly behind them).

The sounds are made in turn, without any precise order or side of presentation. The object is to demonstrate two convincing high and two low frequency responses.

The test sounds **must be quiet**, i.e. less than 40 dB[1] on a sound-level meter. This means that with the meter set at 40 there should be no deflection of the needle.

The sounds

- Arousal stimuli (cup and spoon, squeaker, musical box, etc.) are sometimes used to get the child's attention; but these sounds contain a wide mix of frequencies and therefore their value is limited.
- High frequency: Nuffield rattle, gently rolled at 1 foot from ear, or Manchester rattle gently rolled at 3 feet, and 'sss' as in bus (*not* forced hiss).
- Low frequency: 'oooo' as in shoe; hummed, *not* whispered.
- Warble tones; 0.5 KHz, 1, 2, 4 KHz; produced by an electronic device. (Check recommended test distance for the warbler you are using.) Warblers have the advantage of fixed intensity of sound—you cannot cheat!

[1] If the test sounds are instead presented at 45 dB, the test becomes less sensitive, i.e. it may miss mild degrees of hearing loss but it becomes more specific, i.e. there will be less false positive results and therefore fewer unnecessary referrals. This change in technique may prove to be useful but has not yet been adequately investigated.

The response

To **pass** the child must respond reliably to high and low sounds on both sides. A head turn to seek for the sound is the only positive response which can be passed by screeners. The distractor is responsible for deciding if the child has responded or if what was seen was just a random movement.

Any outcome other than that described above is an indication to **re-test** 6 weeks later, or to refer if there are special circumstances, e.g. parent already concerned or unlikely to return for second test.

Some babies, particularly those who have a hearing loss, are visually very alert and are constantly looking around the room. This is an increasing problem as the baby gets older and is one of the reasons why testing is easier at 7 than at 10 months (p. 170).

Carry out a **no-sound trial** in which the distractor removes stimulation but the tester does not make any sound; observe whether the baby turns during the period of silence. If he does, this may be a warning that previous responses have been unreliable.

Common problems

The most difficult aspects of the test are:

- To control the baby's attention for long enough to complete the test.
- To distinguish between random movements and true responses.
- To avoid false positive turning responses.
- To keep the test sounds quiet enough; a sound-level meter should be used to measure each sound to which the baby responds, preferably for every test, but certainly while one is gaining experience. It is surprisingly difficult to keep the intensity of the sound stimuli as low as 35 dB. There is always a temptation to raise the intensity of sounds in order to elicit a response from the baby or to overcome distracting background noise.

The failed screening test

If the baby does not respond consider the possible reason:

- Until you have proved otherwise, you must assume that the child has a hearing loss.
- Your technique may be inadequate.
- The baby may be in an unsuitable behavioural state.
- The room may be too noisy.
- If good responses are obtained when the sounds are made slightly louder, the cause may be a transient middle ear problem, and this diagnosis would be supported by a history of recent colds or earache. In this situation, it is reasonable to retest the baby in 6 weeks' time.
- If the baby does not respond even when louder sounds are presented, or if the parent already suspected a hearing loss before the screening test was performed, immediate referral is preferred.
- Difficulty in localizing the sound accurately may be due to a mild hearing loss. Secretory otitis in particular seems to impair localization more than one

might expect from the severity of the hearing loss normally found in this condition.

- Children with hemiplegia, hemianopia, or a strong pattern of 'preferred head turning' (p. 169) may also turn more readily to one side than the other.
- Lastly, remember also that global backwardness, autism or visual defect may occasionally present with a failed hearing test. The child either fails to respond at all, shows inconsistent responses or has excessive difficulty in localizing the sound source. These babies are difficult to test; remember that the response time may be prolonged and you should allow adequate time for the baby to turn before repeating the sound stimulus. Do not hesitate to refer 'hard to test' babies.

No baby should have more than two screening tests; if there is still doubt after the second, expert assessment is essential.

Believe your results!

The results of the distraction screening test are often explained away with comments such as 'he wasn't interested' or 'he was tired, bored, etc.'. The child's poor responses are described as 'being unco-operative'. Parents are sometimes told that the child is too young or too difficult to test or that they should wait until the next screening test is due. Such advice is unacceptable. If clinical tests are impossible, one can resort to objective tests (p. 62).

Detection of vision defects

History

Ask the parents whether they have any concerns about the child's vision (*see* questions below).

Questions about vision

Have you any worries about his vision?
Does he look at you and follow with his eyes?
Does he look at his hands?
Does he look at objects or pictures?
Does he recognize you when he sees you?
Does he look at tiny objects, e.g. crumbs on the floor?
Have you ever noticed a squint/cast/wandering or turning eye?

Enquire about family history of vision defects

Squints tend to be more common in some families. If there is a sibling or parent with a squint it may be justified to refer the child for an orthoptic examination and refraction. Squint is most often noticed first by the parents or other family members, but they do not always regard it as important and may not mention it unless specifically asked.

Refractive error also tends to be familial. It is unnecessary to refer infants for refraction solely on grounds of a family history of myopia appearing later in childhood or in adult life. Severe hypermetropia or astigmatism in a first degree relative may however justify referral, if an accessible community orthoptic service is available.

Observe the child's visual behaviour

Does he look at you, his parent, or around the room? Notice how he looks at toys or objects. There is rarely any doubt about a normal child's ability to see.

Inspect the eyes carefully

Look at the eye movements. Wandering or jerking movements are abnormal and are often a sign of poor vision. Nystagmus may be an isolated and often familial condition, or a feature of any disorder causing impaired visual fixation. It is not present at birth but becomes evident in the first few months. Nystagmus in one eye only suggests poor vision in that eye.

Detection of squint

The most efficient way of detecting squint is to **ask the parents**; when parents report a squint they are usually correct, although they do experience the same difficulty as professionals in distinguishing between squint and pseudosquint.

We describe here, for the sake of completeness, the procedures most commonly used for an orthoptic examination, although we doubt that they should be used by anyone other than orthoptists or ophthalmologists unless they have thorough training. The orthoptist spends 3 years learning how to perform and interpret these procedures and they cannot be mastered in half an hour!

Observe whether there is any **head tilt**. This posture is sometimes adopted by the child to compensate for a squint and in itself is sufficient indication for referral. (Remember other possible diagnoses such as sternomastoid tumour, or vertebral anomalies. Very rarely it can be the first sign of a posterior fossa tumour.)

Various forms of squint may be demonstrated by testing **eye movements**.

- If the child is hypermetropic, he may squint when looking at very close objects, so test convergence by bringing the target to within 15 cm of his nose.
- The eyes may fail to move together in a conjugate fashion, or they may separate on upward or downward gaze. Any such abnormality calls for detailed examination.
- Elicit the full range of horizontal, vertical and oblique eye movements by moving a small target in front of the eyes, at about 40 cm distance. A light can be used but a small, interesting toy often holds the child's attention more effectively.
- Small children usually move the whole head rather than the eyes alone when tracking a target so it may be necessary to restrain the head gently with one hand, or ask the mother to do this. The eyes should move smoothly together in all directions. One or two jerks at the extreme lateral range of gaze can be accepted as normal.

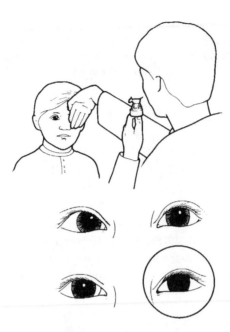

Figure 8.4. The cover tests. These should be performed with a near and a distant target. (Top) Is there a convergent squint in the right eye? (Bottom) When the left eye is covered, the right eye moves outwards to assume fixation. Diagnosis: right manifest convergent squint.

- Persistent **downward deviation** of the eyes is often called the 'sunset sign' because the white rim of sclera above the pupil gives the appearance of the sun going down behind the horizon. It may be a sign of raised intracranial pressure, e.g. in hydrocephalus, and is an indication for urgent referral. However, transient or momentary 'sun-setting' may also be seen in normal babies.
- **Shine a small torch** with a fine beam on the child's eyes from about 40 cm distance. Check whether the reflections are symmetrical in the two eyes. They may not be *central* in the cornea because the eyes may be converged if the child is looking at the light. This is a useful test in cases where you are not sure whether the child has a squint or a pseudosquint.
- The **cover test** is used to determine whether a manifest squint is present. The technique is shown in Figure 8.4. Its most important application in child health surveillance is to distinguish between squint and pseudosquint. It also provides a means of discovering small angle squints which would otherwise be missed, but considerable expertise is required to achieve this.
- The **alternate cover test** is used to elicit a latent squint. Each eye is covered alternately in order to disrupt the fusion mechanisms which normally maintain conjugate gaze. It is even more difficult to interpret than the cover test. There is in any case some doubt about the importance of asymptomatic latent squint.

Orthoptists also use a number of other procedures, for example the base-out prism test and tests of stereopsis (3-D vision). None of these have so far been adopted as screening tests in the UK, but the random dot stereo test has been used in some countries as a screening device for 3-year-olds. It is assumed that if a child can see a three-dimensional pattern, the eyes must be working effectively as a pair and therefore there cannot be any serious eye disease or refractive error. Further work is needed to determine the true value of this screening procedure.

Visual acuity

The measurement of visual acuity is very difficult in children too young to co-operate. Normal visual behaviour and conjugate gaze are the best indicators of satisfactory vision at this age. The ability to detect very small objects can be used to demonstrate visual behaviour.

These tests are known as measures of 'minimum observable' vision. They do not assess the ability to separate adjacent visual stimuli and therefore are not capable of detecting minor degrees of refractive error. Their value is in exploring and recording impaired visual behaviour in infants, which is more often related to general developmental backwardness rather than primary vision dis-orders. Opinions differ as to their role and value as screening tests in child health surveillance.

Normal infants show an obvious interest in objects of 1 or 2 mm diameter by 6 months of age, although they may not be able to grasp them. Tiny cake decorations ('hundreds and thousands') are often used to test this. They should be placed on a dark, flat surface, and if the infant does not immediately show an interest they should be rolled around.* There may be an attempt to poke at the sweets with a finger tip. If you can only retain the child's attention with larger objects, consider whether this reflects developmental immaturity rather than a vision problem.

This procedure may be carried out with each eye patched in turn. If the baby objects violently to one eye being covered but not the other, or there is an obvious difference between the two eyes in the ability to fixate, a unilateral defect should be suspected.

---

* Caution: a visually impaired baby may appear to see a moving object but be unable to fixate his gaze on it when it is stationary.

Health education topics

- **Immunizations:** up to date.

- **Developmental progress:** need for play and language stimulation.

- **Nutrition and diet:** weaning; control of sugar intake.

- **Accident prevention:** child may already be mobile.

Danger	Advice
Scalds—child grabs dangling kettle flex	Safety flexes should be coiled, out of reach.
Falls	Make sure properly restrained in buggies and highchairs. Gate across stairs. Care with baby-walkers.
Poisoning	Keep medicines and household products out of reach (including dishwasher powder).
Cuts	Beware of sharp edges on furniture and toys.
Choking: nuts, sweets, fragments of plastic, pen tops	Keep such objects out of reach.
Severe sunburn (risk of skin tumours in later life)	Sensible precautions (shade, creams, clothing, etc.). Children with fair hair, pale skin and freckles are particularly at risk. The parents should consult the pharmacist and ensure they have a cream with an adequate Sun Protection Factor.

- **Teeth:** careful and regular tooth brushing once teeth appear.

- **Dentist:** has child registered and is (s)he attending at least once annually for a dental check-up and health advice?

1 to 2 years

Contents

This section reviews the normal development of the child between the first and second birthdays and describes some of the common behavioural and developmental problems in that age group. The only routine health contact between 12 and 18 months is for the MMR immunization, but the review recommended between 18 and 24 months is described and the importance of health education and accident prevention at this age is stressed.

Normal development, 12–18 months

Learning and communication

Between 12 and 15 months, play and experimentation with objects occupy the infant for increasingly long periods. He learns about the relationships between objects, putting things in and out of containers or dropping them on the floor. He begins to demonstrate by appropriate use that he understands the function of common objects such as a hairbrush or a cup and spoon (Figure 9.1).

The emergence of spoken language seems to be related to play—delayed language development is often associated with a lack of imaginative play. It is not always easy to define when the first word appears since much depends on the parent's interpretation of the child's vocalization.

By 18 months, the baby has become a toddler; he is usually exploring actively, opening cupboards, climbing on furniture and so on. He understands daily routines and tries to imitate housework and other adult activities. The relationships between shapes and the properties of liquids and solid objects are investigated.

He plays with miniature toys, for example dolls or cars, but the activities performed with them are still fragmentary and he does not yet act out detailed sequences with them. He shows very strong attachments to his care-givers and may still be wary of strangers, although this varies considerably; some toddlers make friends very easily.

It is normal for a child to pass through a phase of mouthing objects and throwing them away ('casting') but this should be a transient phase. Casting does not usually persist beyond 18 months. If casting (other than in a temper tantrum) or persistent indiscriminate mouthing of objects continues beyond the age of 2, this is a worrying sign suggestive of some developmental problem.

Figure 9.1. Definition by use.

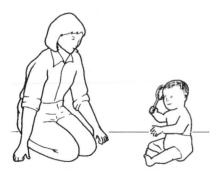

Motor development

Age 12–14 months

- The precise stage at which a toddler walks alone varies with his personality and physical make-up. This is usually between 12 and 15 months, but may vary by several months earlier or later.
- Independent mobility is more important to the child than the method used.
- For many children crawling remains their chosen method for a prolonged period. Walking is no more important to the toddler than any other skill which gives him control over his world, e.g. manipulation, communication or socialization.

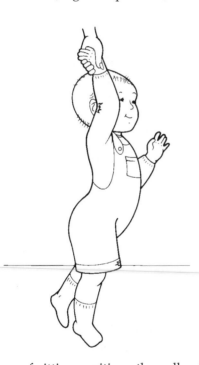

Mobility
- The toddler has the ability to crawl, pull up to standing, cruise, return to the floor, push a chair or a truck and an infinite variation or combination of these.
- He will cruise along the furniture, drop to crawling to bridge a gap and rise to standing again at the next piece of furniture.
- He will walk with one hand held.
- He may rise to standing in free space without the support of furniture. His balance is hazardous!
- He may drop from standing to sitting or crawling in free space.
- He adopts numerous varieties of sitting positions thus allowing himself to get close to his toys, e.g. side-sitting with legs wind-swept to one side or sitting on heels (bunny style).
- He bends down from standing to retrieve a fallen toy.
- He hitches along the floor on his bottom.
- He can move from place to place while hoarding objects in his hands, e.g. crawls around with a brick in each hand.
- He experiments with his body in relationship to objects—crawls under chairs and tables, sits up and bumps his head, climbs up into chairs and onto tables.

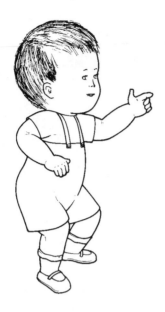

Grasp and manipulation
- Can grasp with almost adult precision but release is still not fully developed.

- Can now release an object in an intended direction, but it takes time and effort.
- Plays with objects and containers.

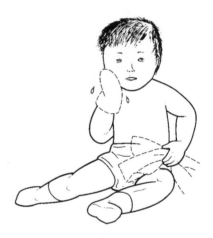

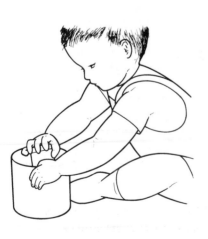

- Enjoys fitting things together.
- Places round shapes into posting box.
- Attempts to build cube tower—places brick on top of brick but fails to release with precision.
- By 13 months can grasp two cubes in one hand simultaneously.

Age 15–18 months

- The toddler has adopted walking as his most usual means of mobility.
- He uses a wide-based gait to increase his stability and will retain this for several months, returning to it when attempting demanding physical tasks.
- Release of objects has become sophisticated, enabling him to engage in building, throwing and posting games.

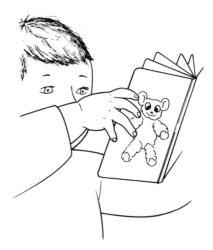

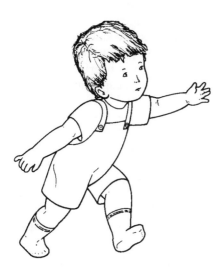

Mobility
- Walks alone on a wide-based gait.
- Rarely falls.
- Attempts to run but knees remain stiff and feet flat on floor.
- Climbs stairs on all fours or walks up with one hand held, the other on rail or stair.
- Descends stairs by hitching on bottom or sliding down on stomach.
- Kneels upright unaided.
- Moves with increasing fluency between standing and squatting and squatting and standing.

Grasp and manipulation
- Balance now adequate to free hands for manipulation.
- Release of objects is well developed.
- Places rings over a post.
- Builds tower of two cubes.
- Manoeuvres cubes into post box.
- Throws ball to adult.
- Carries toys for most of day, tucked under arm.
- Turns pages of books.

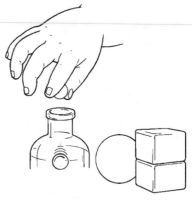

- Scribbles spontaneously, mostly circular but some vertical strokes.

Normal development, 18–24 months

Learning and communication

The pace of **language acquisition** varies enormously—the normal 18-month-old child may have no words or as many as 200. Some will start to join words at or before this age. Nearly all 18-month-olds can understand some words and many can respond to simple commands containing two information words, e.g. 'put the car on the table'.

Attention at this age is said to be single channel. This means that the toddler, once he is immersed in an interesting activity, is unable to continue playing while simultaneously absorbing spoken instructions or suggestions offered by demonstration. The ability to interact in this more mature fashion emerges between 18 and 36 months and is associated with increasing social poise, self-confidence and independence (*see* p. 212). The difference between children of these ages is very striking. The 18-month-old child is still a baby in many respects, whereas the 3-year-old often gives the impression that he is ready for school.

It is possible for a child to have severe delay in language development yet understand the rules of social behaviour and the concept of play very clearly. The clearest example of this is seen in the late-diagnosed partially hearing child and indeed such a pattern of development should always raise a suspicion of hearing loss. More commonly, however, one finds that the child who has slow language development is also immature in the development of attention control, the acquisition of social skills and the emergence of imaginative play.

The process of development can be retarded or facilitated by the **experiences** to which the child is exposed (*see* p. 210). The continued involvement of the caregiver offers encouragement and security. The child's play and exploration can be extended by interventions at appropriate moments, while nevertheless allowing the child to make his own discoveries whenever possible.

Language acquisition is thought to be accelerated by strategies widely used by parents, including expansions and repetitions of the child's brief utterances, giving a more adult model for him to copy; the use of deliberately slow clear speech with a slightly raised pitch or register holds the attention of young children more effectively; and the amount of time devoted to conversation between adult and child is also important.

Although such strategies are associated with more rapid language acquisition, their importance should not be exaggerated. The learning of language seems to be a very robust function in the normal infant. It is unsafe to attribute delayed language development to social or environmental deprivation without first excluding other possible causes.

It should also be remembered that in other cultures, social styles of child rearing may differ from those of white, middle-class professionals. These must not be regarded as abnormal or inferior and if intervention is offered it is important to avoid any hint of judgement or criticism.

Motor development

Age 18–24 months

- By 2 years the toddler has become a physically confident, ambulant child.
- He has an increasing repertoire of mobility and dexterity with which to explore his world.
- The physical skills which he acquired in the first 18 months of life form the basis of all his future refinement of movement.

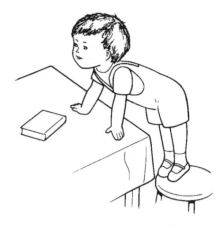

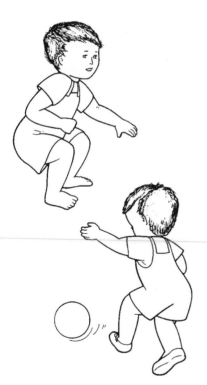

Mobility
- Climbs up stairs with two feet on each step, hand on rail much of the time (he is returning to three points of balance because the task is risky).
- Runs fast and with flexibility of knees and ankles. Changes direction.
- Kicks a ball without falling over. Jumps with both feet together.
- Can bend to retrieve a toy and play for long periods in either squatting or semi-squatting position (half way between standing and squatting).
- Sits in long-sitting (with legs straight out in front) for long periods looking at book or playing with doll on lap.
- Sits astride a tricycle and paddles it along—takes little interest in the pedals.

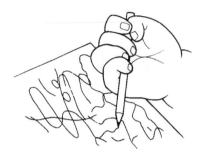

Grasp and manipulation
- Increased movement of wrists and rotation of forearms.
- Now opens and shuts doors, twisting handle.
- Puts on socks.
- Builds tower of six cubes.
- Turns individual pages of book.
- Starts to join large Lego-type bricks.
- Places objects in precise positions constructing neat rows and lines.
- Draws vertical and horizontal strokes.
- Places and manoeuvres simple jigsaw pieces.

- Uses non-dominant hand to steady objects.
- Starting to manoeuvre objects within hand—no longer puts them down to turn them around—may use body to assist.
- Emerging use of individual fingers to assist in manipulation.

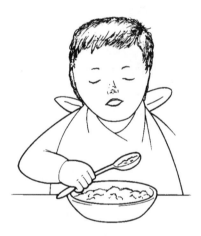

Growth and growth disorders

Parents are more likely to worry about short stature than about excessive growth in height. There should be no hesitation in referring short children. It is acceptable to take two height measurements over a 12 month period *provided that they are accurate enough to be used for subsequent assessment*, but if after this there is still any concern or doubt, the child should be referred for expert opinion. Children with hormonal deficiencies need treatment as early as possible. Each year that passes without appropriate replacement therapy represents some loss in final adult height.

A common observation in conditions causing growth impairment is that the child is not growing out of his trousers or shoes. A question about this can be used as a 'screening' test.

Occasionally parents may be concerned about children (usually daughters) who are growing quickly and becoming abnormally tall (p. 192)—they should be referred at once.

Measuring height

Supine length is measured up to the age of 2: **standing height** thereafter. Standing height is about 0.5 cm less than supine length. This accounts for the kink in the height chart at age 2. Standing height can vary by at least 1 cm during the day.

Obtain a routine measurement of *height* as soon as possible after the age of 18 months, though it can be difficult to get a good measurement before the age of 3.

Accurate measurements are essential. Sticks mounted on scales are unreliable. The Oxford or Middlesex screening charts can be used, but the current best buy for primary care clinics is the Minimeter (available from the Child Growth Foundation). For those who want a more permanent and more robust device, the Magnimetre is recommended.

Measuring procedure

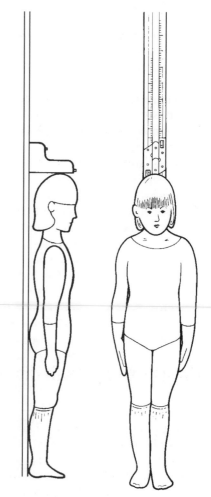

- Remove the child's shoes.
- Ask him to stand with heels against wall or plate.
- Ask an assistant to hold the feet on the ground, so that the child's heels do not rise when you ask him to stand up straight.
- Make sure the child is standing straight. Press the thighs and pelvis gently backwards against the surface of the wall or measuring device.
- Ensure that the upper margin of the auditory meatus is in a horizontal line with the angle of the orbit.
- Steady the child with support under the angle of jaw but do not try to stretch him upwards.
- Measure with your eye in line with the scale to avoid parallax errors.
- Plot on chart.

See Figure 9.2.

Figure 9.2. The Magnimetre.

Height measurements **must be plotted on a suitable chart**, with correction for prematurity if needed. Plot the measurements with care; your chart may one day be required by a specialist colleague or even by a court and wrongly plotted measurements do little for your professional reputation!

New charts were released in autumn 1993 and should now be used in preference to older versions. In case of difficulty, contact the Child Growth Foundation.

No exact rules can be offered for the interpretation of height measurements. It is easier to decide whether or not there is likely to be a significant problem when three or four measurements are available over a period of time. The following guidelines may be helpful:

- Any child whose height is below the 0.4 centile without adequate previous explanation should be fully assessed and usually investigated. Only one child in 250 is this small.
- If parents are clearly worried about the child's height, find out why. Usually they have noticed that he is smaller than his peers, that he is not growing out of his trousers and/or shoes, or that he simply looks small. Parents seldom consult their doctor about short stature until they have observed the child for some time, and they usually make their own decisions about whether their own stature is sufficient explanation! In this situation, it is often better to refer for specialist advice straight away. With the increasing interest in the use of growth hormone for children with relatively mild growth impairment, monitoring of growth should be undertaken in a specialist clinic to facilitate an early decision about treatment.
- If possible growth impairment has been detected at the day nursery or school, find out whether the parents are worried. Check their heights. Then decide with them whether to (a) measure again in 12 months time or (b) refer for specialist advice.
- If measurements are taken less than 12 months apart, or the equipment or measuring technique are inaccurate, interpretation is difficult or impossible.
- The commonest reason for a child to be between the 0.4 and the 2nd centile is that s/he has short parents. A better way of adjusting the child's height for parental height is being developed; meanwhile, as a rule of thumb it is unusual for parents who are both average or above average height to have a child who is below the 2nd centile.
- Any child who has been measured regularly for any reason and whose height crosses two or more centile bands in the pre-school years or more than one centile band between the ages of five and eight is exhibiting an unusual growth pattern that needs explanation. Nevertheless many children with subsequently proven growth disorders do not fulfil these criteria. If there are other reasons to be concerned they should be fully assessed.
- Short stature in association with other problems, notably dysmorphic syndromes, or with *any* additional signs or symptoms, is of course more likely to be pathological and merits referral.
- Ascertain the local guidelines on growth monitoring.

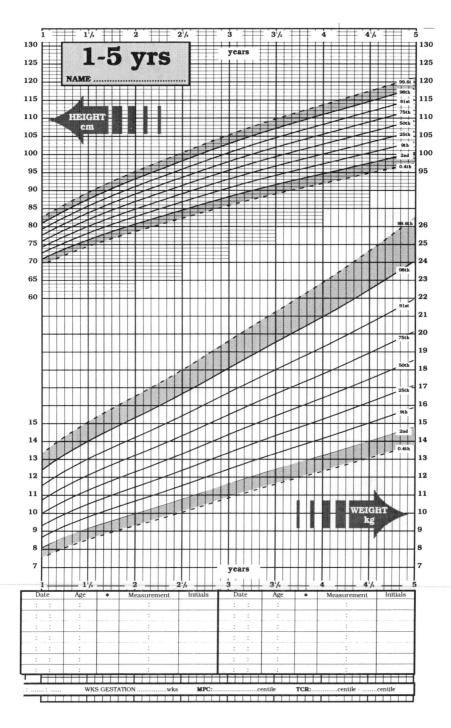

Figure 9.3a. Boys height and growth assessment chart.
(Also available for ages 0–1 years and 5–18 years.)

Reproduced with kind permission from the Child Growth Foundation, 2 Mayfield Avenue, London W4 1PW (Telephone 0181-994-7625).

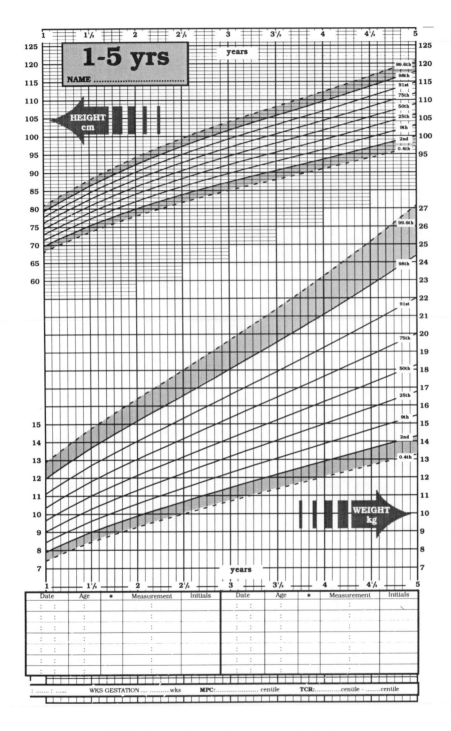

Figure 9.3b. Girls height and growth assessment charts.
(Also available for ages 0–1 years and 5–18 years.)

Reproduced with kind permission from the Child Growth Foundation, 2 Mayfield Avenue, London W4 1PW (Telephone 0181-994-7625).

Growth velocity

Until recently, this was thought to be more useful than a single measurement but it is now clear that growth velocity does not perform well as a method of screening for growth disorders. Careless measurements can result in errors of 2 cm or more but even experts have unavoidable measurement errors and when these are compounded over successive occasions, a cumulative error of 2 cm can occur over a 12 month period. This may represent the difference between normal and abnormal growth velocity.

Important causes of short stature

Genetic and familial

By definition 2 per cent of children are below the 2nd centile in height (i.e. more than 2 SDs from the mean). Most of them are normal short children and in many cases the parents are also short. When the height is below the 0.4 centile line there is more likely to be a specific cause.

Intrauterine growth retardation

This is a common cause of short stature. Although children who have lost weight acutely in the last few weeks of pregnancy often catch up completely in height and weight, those who have suffered prolonged malnutrition may remain small. A minority of these babies have some recognizable dysmorphic syndrome.

Malnutrition

This is usually associated in developed countries with psychosocial deprivation (*see* p. 82); this may lead to impairment of linear growth as well as failure to gain weight. More rarely, under-nutrition occurs when health food enthusiasts offer their children highly unsuitable diets, with too much fibre and insufficient energy content (*see* p. 23).

Endocrine causes

The most important treatable causes of short stature are **hypothyroidism** and **growth hormone deficiency**. Although congenital hypothyroidism is detected in the neonatal period in most cases, juvenile cases can occur sporadically through-out childhood and short stature may be the only sign. Growth hormone deficiency can also present at any age; it should be detected as early as possible in order to obtain the best results from treatment.

Turner's syndrome

This is easily overlooked in infancy and early childhood. The well-known features of this condition, such as webbing of the neck, shield-shaped chest and wide carrying angle at the elbow are not invariably present, although most of these girls have spoon-shaped fingernails.

The short stature, which may be the only clue to the diagnosis in childhood, may not be apparent until 6 or 7 years of age. Special growth charts are available for girls with Turner's syndrome. Note that in early childhood the height and height velocity may be within normal limits. Early diagnosis and referral to a growth clinic are desirable, and the availability of new approaches to treatment may improve the prognosis for adult height.

Other causes

Short stature can occasionally be the sole presenting feature of chronic disease such as **renal failure, inflammatory bowel disease (mainly Crohn's) and coeliac disease**.

Various **chondrodystrophies**, although individually very rare, should be considered. Many of these conditions are diagnosed at birth, but in some the disproportion in length between trunk and limbs which later becomes obvious is not present in infancy and short stature is the only feature. Early diagnosis is important because of genetic counselling and also because new treatment possibilities are under investigation.

The causes of **tall stature** include: genetic and familial factors, Marfan's syndrome, Klinefelter's syndrome, thyrotoxicosis, growth hormone excess, precocious puberty, etc. Tallness is a rare complaint and one for which parents usually seek advice, particularly where daughters are concerned. Specialist investigation is usually necessary and referral should be offered **as soon as the problem is presented**, as early treatment is essential if the aim is to reduce the adult height by any significant amount.

Summary of review between 18 and 24 months

- Review:
  - Family concerns
  - Child's progress
    Language
    Motor function.
- Discuss behaviour and behavioural problems.
- Ask if concerns about hearing or vision.
- Ask about growth in height and measure height if possible.
- Consider possibility of iron deficiency.
- Health education topics.

Review between 18 and 24 months

Children in this age group are particularly difficult to evaluate in a clinic or consulting room and it is often better to make a home visit. When resources are scarce, parents who are known to be experienced and competent may be contacted by letter or telephone and invited to report to the health visitor if there are any concerns.

Content of the review

- A **physical examination** is *not* normally included as part of the check at this age.
- Measure the **height** (length if under the age of 2) if the child is sufficiently co-operative to allow accurate measurement. Check the weight if any reason to be concerned.
- Consider the possibility of child neglect or abuse if there is evidence of failure to thrive, excessive bruising, delay in development and particularly in language acquisition.
- Confirm that the child is **walking** and that the **gait is normal**. Ninety-seven per cent of children are walking by 18 months.
- No attempt should be made to screen for vision or hearing defects except by simple observation and by asking the parents appropriate questions. If there is any reason to be concerned, refer to the second-tier clinic (hearing) or orthoptist or eye clinic (vision).
- Review **language** and **motor development** with the parents.
- Although most children are beginning to produce some words and to show more definite evidence of understanding language, the variation is too wide and evaluation too difficult to recommend that one should try to screen for language disorders. However, if the parents voice any concerns these must be taken seriously.
- Often the main concerns at this age are to do with **management issues**, such as tantrums, sleep disturbances, food fads or poor appetite, toilet training battles and so on. Some parents value advice on how to deal with these, others may simply want reassurance that they are responding correctly.
- There is a high incidence of **iron deficiency** at this age, which may be a cause of irritability, developmental and behavioural problems as well as anaemia. Some GPs offer a screening service for iron deficiency anaemia in this age group (*see* p. 22).

Referral of speech and language problems

- If the parents are worried, a consultation with a speech therapist and a hearing test should be suggested.
- If a health visitor, social worker or playgroup leader express concern, but the parent is not apparently worried, the situation is more difficult. If in doubt, ask advice from a community paediatrician
- Do not accept the following as 'explanations' for delay in speech and language development:
  - Boys are always slower than girls.
  - Second children are slower than first.
  - Exposure to more than one language.
  - Twins have a secret language.
  - He is lazy.

Common movement problems

- It is surprisingly rare in the UK that late walking is the presenting complaint in this age group. There are two likely reasons for this: either the child has already been diagnosed as having some neurological or developmental disorder, or the parents decide not to seek referral because they have a family history of late walking. Nevertheless, it is wise to look carefully at any child who is not walking at 18 months.

- Unilateral **dislocation of the hip** will give rise to a limp and is unlikely to be overlooked. Bilateral dislocation is associated with a delay in walking in some children but the majority walk at the normal time. The gait is waddling and there is a marked lumbar lordosis. *However, many children with late presenting CDH have other features whose significance is easily overlooked*—walking on tiptoe, short leg, failure of one foot to touch the ground in the baby-walker, difficulty in crawling, a 'funny walk', dragging one leg, inability to sit astride a bicycle or adult's knee, falling to one side, delay in walking, pain on walking, and grating or clicking sensations felt by the adult when holding the child.

- **Bottom shufflers**; these babies are rather floppy, slow to sit, dislike being placed in a prone position, tend to stick their legs out in front of them when held vertical, instead of placing their feet down and taking weight, and shuffle on their bottoms instead of walking. They walk late, sometimes as late as 30 months. There is often a positive family history of shuffling. If you do not know about it, you may wrongly diagnose cerebral palsy or muscle disease. But babies with these disorders may also shuffle!

- **Tiptoe walking** is an unusual pattern of development. In most cases it is intermittent and the feet can be placed flat on the floor. The balance is often remarkably good—it has to be to permit the ballerina gait characteristic of these toddlers. Occasionally the heelcords are very tight and although spontaneous resolution is the rule, a physiotherapy assessment is reassuring to both doctor and parent. If there is any additional feature such as weakness or a family history of any neuromuscular disorder, full paediatric evaluation is essential.

- Observe the gait carefully: any boy who has an **abnormal gait**, evidence of weakness on stairs or steps, or does not learn to run within a few months of starting to walk, or who has difficulty in stooping and recovering the upright position, should be referred for a blood CPK test to exclude **Duchenne dystrophy**.

- Hand preference may be appearing by this age but its absence is not abnormal.

- A slight **tremor or shakiness** of the hands while playing with toys is normal. It may persist for a year or more and is more obvious under stress. Unless it is getting worse or there are other signs of abnormality, it is almost certainly innocent and should not be regarded as a sign of ataxia.

Thinking about language development

Most of the children with serious problems of language development are first referred by the parents; their main difficulty is that professionals often offer spurious reassurance instead of arranging a thorough assessment. In some cases, parents may wait well into the third year before taking action; when they do present the child for advice, they are usually fairly certain that there is something wrong.

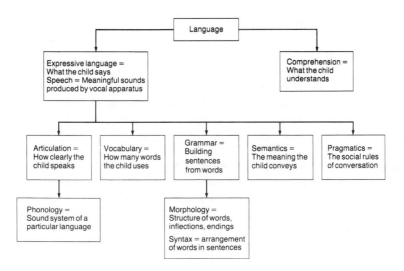

Figure 9.4. Terms used by speech therapists.

There is often concern about the effects of a deprived and under-stimulating environment on language acquisition. As part of the overall spectrum of inadequate child rearing, delay and impoverishment in language development and usage is very common. It is important to anticipate and recognize this situation, and where possible to intervene. Although the language delay may be the most obvious feature, such children are also likely to be deficient in other skills; their ability to concentrate, to originate ideas, to interact with other children and so on.

If any lasting change is to be brought about in such families, it is not sufficient to identify 'speech delay' as an isolated problem or to 'treat' it by referral to a speech therapist. A more global approach is needed such as that developed in Bristol by Dr Walter Barker. There is mounting evidence that a well-planned and continuing programme of intervention that involves both parent and child can bring about worthwhile gains in a variety of skills, not merely in language development. Such a programme may have long-term benefits which can be identified even ten years later.

Clinical implications

It is *not* necessary to carry out a detailed evaluation of language development in every child. But a knowledge of normal language acquisition can be used to teach parents how *they* can help the child's development and recognize problems themselves. Parents need to know what to expect over the next 12–18 months.

It is easier to understand the process of learning to speak if you are familiar with the various terms used to describe language (*see* Figure 9.4).

Observation

- Ask the parents about the child's **use of words** and **understanding of instructions**. Observe how the child responds to any comments or remarks made to him by the parent, and to any extraneous noises in the room.

- Watch how the child **plays with toys**.
- Note persistence of **mouthing** and **casting** (pointless indiscriminate throwing away of objects, which usually indicates that the child does not understand their function or symbolic meaning) which at this age should have disappeared or at most be only occasional and brief.
- It is useful to have a box of toys with six or eight items (brush, spoon, chair, doll, cup, ball, car). Check with the parent whether each is familiar. Put them on the table one by one. You can ask the child 'What's that one?' once for each toy, pausing briefly and telling him yourself if he does not respond. Invite him to name the body parts on the doll. Explain how the child demonstrates his understanding by using the object even if he cannot name it.
- Test the ability to **link two ideas**. For instance, ask him to put the doll on the chair, give the brush to mummy. Remember that it is natural for a small child to place objects in containers, so the ability to put a toy in a box does not necessarily confirm that the child has understood the instruction.

Health education topics

- **Immunization:** up to date.

- **Nutrition and dental care:** are any teeth obviously decayed—if necessary refer to a dentist.

- **Accident prevention:**

Danger	Advice
Road safety	Keep under constant control whenever near roads. Use pedestrian safety harness if possible.
Falls	Restrict access to balconies and beware of low windows. Lock them if possible.
Drowning	Keep under constant control when near water. Drownings in pools and ponds are more likely to happen at times of disruption to the normal routine, for instance on special occasions such as weddings, or on outings to parks or garden centres.
Poisons	Remember some garden plants are highly poisonous. Medicine containers are at best child-**resistant**, not child-**proof**.

- **Developmental needs.** Mixing with other children, learning to play with them and to share possessions, playgroups and nurseries, language stimulation.

- **Behavioural difficulties.** Disturbance of sleep, eating battles, toilet training, tantrums—all *very* common. If you intend to do more than offer sympathy, learn some simple psychological principles and techniques.

- By 21 months, 75 per cent of children can point to a named body part and **follow a single instruction**. The parent may be able to give equivalent examples, e.g. 'Where's your nose?', 'Take the shoes to daddy'. Between 80 and 90 per cent of children aged 2 can understand at least one such request.
- The more advanced child will be able to identify pictures, and will be able to point to pictures that indicate actions such as running, jumping or crying, e.g. 'Which girl is running?'
- Ascertain the child's **social skills** by asking the parents, supported by observation as necessary. By the age of 2, most children can use a spoon and a cup adequately without spilling, can remove several items of clothing, try to put on their shoes, appreciate the functions of a book so that pages are turned singly, and play for a short time alone.
- It is normal for the 2-year-old to be aggressive in defence of his possessions and to play alongside rather than *with* other children.
- Show the parent how children can be helped to develop their language and play abilities.

Interpretation

Although 80 to 90 per cent of 18-month-old children have at least a few words, delay in beginning to speak is of less concern at this age *provided that* there is evidence of comprehension.

A child who has less than six words at age 2 is certainly very slow, although not necessarily abnormal. The parents may recognize the child's frustration at being unable to communicate his ideas or wants, often expressed as tantrums; this problem reaches its peak incidence early in the third year. There is more likely to be a **serious problem** if:

- The child is very silent.
- There is persistent continuous dribbling.
- The child has substantial problems with chewing and swallowing.
- There is other evidence of a movement disorder, such as floppiness or clumsiness.
- The child does not show any desire to communicate by any means. If by the age of 20 months a child is neither 'pretending' nor pointing to indicate needs, s/he is unlikely to be interested in what adults are trying to point out to them. These features correlate with later diagnoses of autism and communication disorder and merit referral to a child development team. It is not yet clear whether the natural history of these problems can be altered but parents can learn to handle their unusual child much more effectively.
- A child of 18 months with little or no **understanding** of simple familiar words and phrases spoken by the parent, or a 2-year-old unable to identify any of your toys or objects correctly should be regarded with concern.
- Usually, the child whose speech and comprehension are delayed in this age group is also somewhat immature in other respects, notably in play, concentration and attention control. The child who cannot maintain his attention on any task is at increased risk of having persistent developmental and behavioural difficulties.

If you see a child with substantial difficulty in comprehension, but who has well developed play and social competence, the diagnosis is **hearing loss** until proved otherwise. Any child who does present in this age range with concern about lack of speech or understanding of speech, must have a **hearing test** before any conclusions can be drawn about the cause of the delay. There is no screening test suitable for use in this age group. Any doubt about hearing is an indication for referral to the second-tier audiology clinic.

Vision tests

There are no suitable screening tests. Refer any child whose parents have worries about squint or vision defects.

Frequent falls and funny feet

Two common and often related complaints in children who have just begun to walk are that the child falls too often and that the feet 'do not look right'. The most common problems are **intoeing**, **outtoeing**, **metatarsus adductus** (banana-shaped feet), **knock knees**, **bow legs** and **flat feet**. Correct diagnosis of these usually benign problems and adequate explanation and reassurance for the parents depend on an understanding of normal growth patterns in the lower limbs.

The femur and tibia spiral as they grow and therefore, during growth, the feet may not point the same way as the legs. They may point inward (**intoeing**), so that each can catch on the other leg as the child runs. If they point outwards (**outtoeing**), they may catch on obstacles, again leading to more falls than expected.

Clinical assessment

- Establish if there is a family history of serious bone disease or any evidence of progressive deterioration. In most cases neither is present and the parents can confirm that although the child falls frequently, he is walking, running and climbing and becoming progressively more expert at these skills. If there is any doubt about these points, consider the possibility of **muscular dystrophy** (*see* p. 194) or **cerebral palsy**.
- Watch the child walking and running. If there is any limp or asymmetry of gait, or any hint of weakness, specialist referral is advisable.
- Even if the child has been screened previously, congenital dislocation of the hips can be missed, particularly if the condition is bilateral. This results in a waddling gait with protruding buttocks. With the child supine, flex the hips and look for limitation of abduction. Obtain an X-ray if there is any doubt.
- Always look at the base of the spine for abnormalities characteristic of **occult spinal dysraphism** (*see* p. 134).
- Once any serious problems have been excluded, take a more careful look at the child's feet and legs.

Intoeing

This can be associated with one or more of the following:

- **Femoral neck anteversion**. In infancy, the angle between the femoral neck and head, and the femoral shaft, is different from that observed in the older child and adult. Instead of pointing inwards, the head and neck point forwards. As the child grows, the femur spirals until the adult position is reached. If the child starts to walk while the femoral heads are still pointing forwards, the child rotates the leg inwards as he walks, in order to maintain the position of the femoral head firmly in the acetabulum. The child therefore walks with the knee-caps facing each other and the feet pointing inwards.

    This can be demonstrated to the parents by placing the child prone (Figure 9.5, a,b,c) and showing that the legs can be rotated inwards often to 90°, whereas the outward or external rotation is greatly reduced (Figure 9.5, d). This apparently alarming 'deformity' almost always resolves with growth, usually by age 8 or 9 years, and no treatment should be given or suggested.

- **Tibial torsion**. The tibia spirals as it grows in the same way as the femur. If the growth and rotation of the tibia is out of step with that of the femur, the foot may be either inwardly or outwardly rotated. Inward rotation of the foot is associated with internal tibial torsion and leads to intoeing. It is usually associated with outward curving of the tibia, giving an apparent bow-leg appearance. Clinical assessment is rather more difficult than in the case of the thigh. It is necessary to assess the thigh–foot angle as shown in Figure 9.6, a,b,c.

- **Metatarsus adductus (varus)**. Some children have feet with an inward curve between the heel and the toes, giving the foot the appearance of a banana (Figure 9.7). The condition is distinguished from clubfoot by the normal position and appearance of the heel. In most cases the deformity is minor and corrects spontaneously. The child need only be referred if the deformity is severe.

Outtoeing

Parents often become alarmed when they observe that as the child stands and begins to walk, the feet turn out, sometimes to nearly 90°. Examination (Figure 9.5, e) shows that the hips are externally rotated and internal rotation is much reduced (the opposite situation to that shown in Figure 9.5, d). Spontaneous correction occurs in most cases and no treatment is needed.

Knock knees and bow legs

A mild degree of bow legs (genu varus) is commonly seen up to the age of 2 (Figure 9.8, a) and between 2 and 4 knock knees (genu valgus) is a normal finding (Figure 9.8, b). The degree of rotation of the hips should be checked because internal rotation of the hips leads to the appearance of knock knees.

The extent of the deformity is easily determined. For bow-legs, the ankles are brought together until they just touch and the distance between the knees is

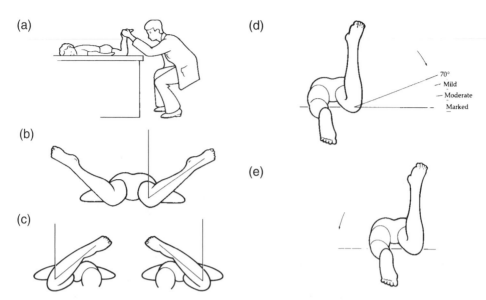

(a)

(b)

(c)

(d)

70°
Mild
Moderate
Marked

(e)

Figure 9.5. (a) Assessment of hip rotation—child lies prone (b) Assessment of internal rotation (c) Assessment of external rotation–each hip is checked separately (d) Increased internal rotation (e) Increased external rotation.

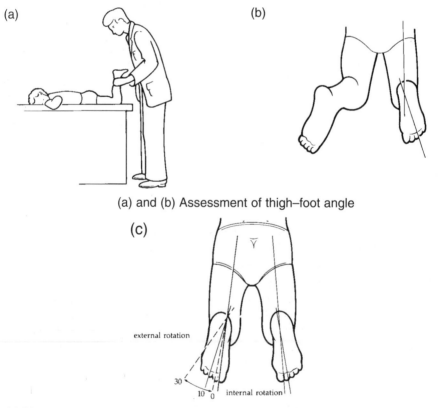

(a)

(b)

(a) and (b) Assessment of thigh–foot angle

(c)

external rotation

30

10 0 internal rotation

(c) Normal range of thigh–foot angle is 0–30° of external rotation with a mean of 10°

Figure 9.6. Tibial torsion.

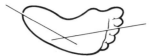

Figure 9.7. Metatarsus adductus (varus).*

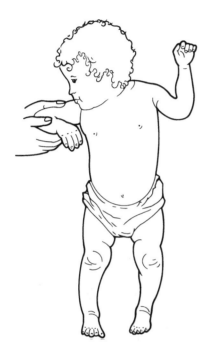

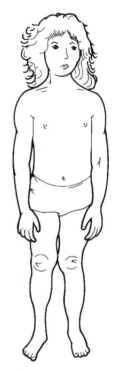

Figure 9.8a. A mild degree of bow legs (genu varus).*

Figure 9.8b. Knock knees (genu valgus).*

measured. To assess the degree of knock knees, the knees are brought together until the inside of the knees just touch and the feet are pointing straight forward. The distance between the malleoli of the ankles is measured and recorded. Up to 6 or 7 cm is generally accepted as normal in each case.

Rickets is only rarely the cause of knock knees or bow legs, and other diseases causing these deformities are even less common. If the measurement is steadily increasing over time or if the child is unwell or miserable in any way, or has a poor diet (*see* Chapter 2) he should be referred.

* Reproduced with kind permission from *The Pediatric Clinics of North America*, November 1977, Volume 24, Number 4, published by W. B. Saunders.

Other foot problems

Parents may become anxious about **flat feet**, particularly if they had supposedly 'suffered' from flat feet in childhood themselves. The child should be asked to stand on tiptoe. If the arch is seen to form normally when he does this the foot is normal and no treatment is required.

High arched or 'cavus' feet, and **clawing of the toes**, are more likely to be abnormal and may have a neurological cause; such children should be referred.

Over-riding of the fifth toe over the fourth is common and though not serious can be a troublesome problem to treat. Attractive simple solutions such as strapping do not help, but, if necessary, the toe can be straightened by surgery.

Referral

The child should be referred if any deformity appears to be asymmetrical, deteriorating, or unusually severe. Often parental concern will only be eliminated by a specialist opinion, even if the primary care staff are confident that the child's physical findings are within the normal range.

Common management problems

Breath-holding

There are two sorts of breath-holding spells: blue and white.

Blue (cyanotic) spells are found in babies and toddlers and are not uncommon, affecting perhaps 5 per cent of all children. They appear to run in families. A typical spell is precipitated by frustration and rage. Furious crying halts at the end of expiration after a few yells. The glottis is then held closed, blocking inspiration. After about 5 seconds cyanosis can be seen and the child loses consciousness. There may be a rigid opisthotonic posture, possibly a few clonic movements. Recovery is swift and complete. Differentiation from epilepsy is made on the basis of a clear precipitant, a clear history of forceful crying before consciousness is lost, and the absence of confusion or drowsiness afterwards.

Consider whether the child is **anaemic**. If so, correction of the anaemia can abolish the behaviour. The mechanism is unknown.

Although parents are traditionally urged to ignore breath-holding spells, this is exceptionally difficult. If it were crucial, many older children and adults would retain the habit; they do not. What parents want to know is whether it is a dangerous habit (it is not), whether it is epilepsy (no) or may turn into it (also no), and how to terminate attacks when they occur.

With respect to the latter, flicking drops of cold water on the baby's face sometimes works. It is not necessary to provide a drenching with a tumblerful.

The condition is benign. There is no risk of anoxic brain damage. Minimal intervention is the order of the day. Anticonvulsants and sedatives are useless. Should the above measures fail, the parents can be told to place the child in a safe place and carry on with what they are doing. At all costs they must avoid being manipulated by the child or becoming anxiously overprotective.

White (pallid) spells are different. Following surprise, pain or mild injury such as bumping the head in a fall while learning to walk, the child falls limp and apnoeic. Robust crying does not precede apnoea, the breath is not clearly held in expiration, nor is cyanosis very prominent. The child's state reflects the effect of high vagal tone with bradycardia or even transient asystole. **An anoxic seizure may follow**. This is aetiologically different from epilepsy since it is a consequence of cerebral ischaemia—words must be carefully chosen when explanations are given to parents so as to avoid unnecessary alarm. Recovery is swift and uneventful unless a seizure has supervened, in which case some drowsiness is common.

It is sensible to check the cardiovascular system clinically but there are no other investigations that are routinely helpful. If there is doubt about the diagnosis, it can be confirmed by an EEG with simultaneous eyeball pressure (although it is difficult to find technicians who will do this).

Treatment is essentially reassurance and advice to the parents to make sure the child comes to no harm during his brief spell of unconsciousness. They should not pick him up during an attack and place him in an upright position because of the risk of compromising cerebral blood flow and precipitating a seizure. No medication is required. The same dangers of overprotection or indulgence as mentioned previously are present. Medical overenthusiasm may foster the development of such parental responses.

A sizeable minority of preschool children with white breath-holding spells will go on in later childhood to fainting in response to pain or surprise. Otherwise the condition is benign and self-limiting within early childhood.

Febrile convulsions

The diagnosis of a first febrile convulsion is supported by the following:

- Child between 6 months and 3 years of age (febrile fits can occur for the first time outside these limits but the diagnosis should be reviewed with extra care).
- High fever, particularly if there is an obvious cause (earache, viral rash, etc.).
- A brief convulsion (less than 10 minutes).
- Child rapidly recovers and has no further fits.
- Family history of febrile fits.

Beware of cases where:

- The child is under 6 months of age.
- There is only a slight fever or none at all.
- There are other major symptoms of illness—e.g. persistent vomiting, severe diarrhoea.
- The fit lasts more than 10 minutes.
- There are repeated fits in the same illness.
- The child does not recover full consciousness or there is continued marked drowsiness.
- Meningitis, encephalitis and meningococcal septicaemia are rare—but they are devastating illnesses. *Always* consider them in any sick child with a fit or unexplained disturbance of consciousness. In young children the absence of neck stiffness does *not* exclude these diagnoses.

Points to remember:

- A first febrile fit is terrifying to the parents—they think the child is dying.
- They will greatly appreciate a visit even if the diagnosis seems obvious.
- True febrile fits have a very benign prognosis.
- Long-term prophylactic anticonvulsants should only be prescribed by a paediatrician and only in exceptional cases.
- For most children, the optimal management is to provide the parents (and if necessary nursery staff) with rectal diazepam (stesolid), 5 mg if under 3 years old, and 10 mg if over 3. Carry some in the emergency bag.
- Fever control by removal of clothes, tepid sponging and paracetamol may help *prevent* febrile fits but will *not* stop them once they have begun.
- White breath-holding attacks can occur in febrile illnesses and are easily mistaken for a febrile fit.

Tantrums

Temper tantrums are a normal feature of development in the preschool years. They become a problem when they are too frequent, too intense, when parents lose their authority over the child and cannot get him to do what they want, or when they fail to subside as the child matures.

Assessment: specific

Establish the ABC of one or two recent tantrums:

A What were the *a*ntecedents to the tantrum.
B What was the *b*ehaviour during the tantrum.
C What were the *c*onsequences which followed the tantrum.

Start with the **B**. What exactly constitutes a tantrum? Novice parents may have an exaggerated view of what ordinary children do. Next establish the **C**. What do they actually do during and after the tantrum. Do not be fobbed off with a claim that they 'ignore' the child—exactly how do they do that? Lastly find out the **A**. What were the immediate precipitants for a given tantrum? Not uncommonly these include the parent having a tantrum at the child or otherwise behaving unreasonably. Few parents will tell you about this spontaneously or early in the consultation, so leave it until after establishing Bs and As for recent specific instances and ask them 'What exactly were you doing just before he started to shout . . .?

Assessment: general

- **General health of child**. Pain or other discomfort, fatigue (usually insufficient sleep).
- **Delayed language development**. Due to the frustration of the child at not being able to communicate his needs. Check hearing.
- **Mental age of child**. A child who is intellectually immature for his age will be slow to grow out of childish practices and slow to learn tolerance, adequate communication, or postponement of gratification.

- **Consistency of parental discipline**. Parents who say one thing one day and another the next (or who disagree between themselves) have muddled and irritated children. Giving in to tantrums encourages them to recur.
- **Example provided by parents or older siblings**. No child who sees his elders and betters having tantrums will learn more acceptable ways of resolving frustration or conflict.
- **Medication**. Benzodiazepines, hypnotics, anticonvulsants and broncho-dilators can all affect mood adversely.
- **Mental state of child**. Preoccupations, distress at playgroup or school, depressed mood or other causes of irritability.

Management

The ABC analysis and the consideration of general factors may give you some guidelines for advice or action.
   In general terms there are four components of management:

- **Avoiding provocation**. This relates to the antecedents. Excitable children will need forewarning of events known to produce tantrums (bedtimes, etc.). Parents may need to learn how to express their wishes clearly and explicitly (saying what they want the child to do rather than telling the child continually what he must not do), not to tease their offspring, and not to set a bad example by throwing tantrums themselves.
- **Withdrawing attention**. There is nothing wrong with the traditional advice to ignore a tantrum; it is just very difficult to put into practice. Simply telling parents to ignore it is not enough. More specific instruction is required. One possibility is for the **parent to remove themselves** from the room where the tantrum is taking place. For instance they could grab a towel and a portable radio and go and have a bath, locking the bathroom door. To take things to such lengths is not always practical and often it is enough just to leave the room without talking to the child and refusing to answer his demands. The child should be left (ignored) for at least 3 minutes or until he starts to calm down, whichever is the sooner. This approach will only apply if the child can safely be left: having a tantrum in the kitchen when pans are on the gas ring means that a toddler cannot be left there.
   Alternatively, the **child is removed** from the room to some uninteresting part of the house such as the hall. The principle is the same as above and is often called 'time out' because the child is put out of the room. Actually all withdrawal of attention represents time out since this is shorthand for 'time out from positive social reinforcement'. A similar time of 3 minutes or until the tantrum begins to calm is indicated.
- **Not giving in**. The child will learn that making demands in aggressive, threatening or histrionic ways is ineffective.
- **Tuition in alternative ways of responding to frustration**. If the child does not have a tantrum, what can he do? This must be discussed with the parent with reference to the example elicited in the assessment. If the answer is that the child should comply with parental demands, then compliance without throwing a tantrum needs to be rewarded by pointed praise ('Well done for not getting cross!') perhaps in combination with a star chart whereby stars are

earned for immediate compliance. Similar principles apply to frustration arising out of, say, motor clumsiness: the child needs to learn sober strategies for coping with frustration and disappointment. These have to be taught by parents who must explain, demonstrate and praise accordingly.

None of these approaches works immediately; they require several weeks to yield satisfactory results. In order to keep up morale and motivation, some form of charting helps. This may be a simple record, day by day, of the number of tantrums. A more informative system is to ask the parent to compile an ABC for each tantrum. This can then be discussed with the parent at weekly appointments. One twist is to ask the parent to enter the A and B *immediately* the tantrum occurs and ask for the record sheet to be kept permanently in a part of the house where tantrums are least likely to occur (such as the parents' bedroom). This has the effect of removing the parent from the child when a tantrum occurs and depriving him of attention.

Tantrums in public places such as supermarkets are more difficult since ignoring becomes impossible. One answer is not to take the child but this may be unavoidable. Usually the tantrum arises out of a mixture of boredom and craving for displayed goods—the check-out queue is the worst place for both. Distracting the child with a toy, book, packet of raisins (press them down inside the box to make them less likely to spill) or, more realistically, a tube of sweets bought *beforehand* is one possibility. An older toddler may be able to hang on to the idea that not getting cross in the shop can be rewarded by being able to choose something from the check-out display at the end. The important principle is preventing the tantrum occurring in the first place and avoiding being coerced into giving into the child because the embarrassment of the tantrum is overwhelming.

Sibling jealousy

There may be some value in distinguishing between the response of a toddler to a new baby brother or sister and the feelings older siblings have towards each other.

With the birth of a younger sibling, for example a sister, a young child may show overt hostility, crafty sadism or regression. On the other hand, he may be neutral or even welcome her. In the case of a negative reaction, the response is not to the baby as a person, it is a response to changes in the parents or altered relationships in the family. The parents may be preoccupied or exhausted, grandparents are primarily interested in the new baby and so forth. She is blamed by her brother for the changes in his world. He may also be jealous of her as an individual but this is not necessarily so.

If sibling jealousy appears as a problem at this stage, it is too late for prevention as advised in so many child care manuals. Certainly there is value in involving the child actively in the preparations for birth and providing him with a doll to care for. By the time the problem is manifest, a different approach is needed.

- The parents should consider what has changed in the older child's world and whether some things can be reinstated. In particular they must ensure they are devoting attention to the child as well as to the baby. They must make time to play and talk to him on his own.

- They can involve the child in baby care: unfolding nappies, choosing clothes, brushing hair, etc. under supervision so that he feels he has an active role in the newly enlarged family.
- When the baby is a little older, her responses to her older brother can be demonstrated so that he can see how she smiles at him.
- The parents should examine their own relationship with the child. Has father backed away from baby care and simultaneously removed himself from child care?

The situation with older children is likely to be different. Siblings may actually dislike each other. There is no law which says that they have to love each other, although it is reasonable to expect the older ones to bear some responsibility for the younger one's safety.

Teasing between siblings is widespread and may reflect power relationships, rivalry for parental attention, or the way in which a younger sibling may remind an older one of how gauche, puny or naïve he was himself at an earlier age. There is no reason why it cannot be treated as a disciplinary issue. If parents are in doubt as to who started it, separate both parties for a short time (15–30 minutes) turning a deaf ear as to protests. It is preferable to run the risk of unfairness than to allow the teasing to continue.

Chronic teasing raises the question as to whether the parents are too pre-occupied to offer the children a satisfactory ration of attention so that there is fierce competition for any parental response, positive or negative. Some parents respond to this by saying, in effect: 'I disapprove of both of you and will have nothing to do with you until you learn to get on together'. This makes things worse. The correct principle is to devote more time to building each child's self-esteem by finding things that they can do which earn them praise and approval, *separate* from each other. These can include helping around the house, small tasks or errands, and constructive or creative play which has an end product worthy of acclaim. All this requires a measure of active involvement of the parent. Leaving small (or large) children together in front of the television for hours on end is a recipe for squabbles.

2 to 5 years

Contents

This section describes the changes in the child's ability to think and play, and the ways in which he masters language and the social rules that govern communication and interaction. The preschool examination is reviewed and health education topics are emphasized. The common problems of behaviour and development are discussed and there is a detailed description of the methods available for their assessment and treatment.

Normal development, 2–5 years

Cognitive development

Cognitive in the narrow sense means 'to do with thinking' and thus involves reasoning, memory and knowledge. It interacts with emotion to produce attitudes, motivation and meaning. Any of these may be significant clinically.

Intelligence

Intelligence is one measure of cognitive capacity. It can be thought of as the ability to derive meaning from experience and apply it to solving problems. Inherited factors, elements which govern general development (such as nutrition), and environment all combine to influence its development. In Western society, genetic factors are particularly influential since gross deprivations of stimulation or nutrition are unlikely. Some specific causes of intellectual handicap in childhood (Down's syndrome, etc.) are well recognized but are not considered here.

A common failing among contemporary middle class parents is an irrational anxiety as to whether they are providing sufficient stimulation for their child's intellectual development. If they are concerned, then they are already doing so. The only danger is that they will try too hard and put the child under unreasonable pressure or bombard him with stimulation which goes right over his head. Reading Shakespeare to a baby will not steep him in the Bard. Stimulation should be at the child's level of understanding, be relevant to his interests (must engage him), and allow for his participation in it as far as possible (be interactive). This means that television can be appropriate when it is providing information but inappropriate when it is producing escapist entertainment.

As a crude rule of thumb, curiosity is an indication of intelligence in the very young child, self-organization in the older. Motor milestones are a poor guide, creativity only a loose indicator, and memory is not very helpful. Speed of learning is virtually synonymous with intelligence. For older children, school performance is usually reliable.

Intelligence can be measured with very reasonable accuracy by a clinical or educational psychologist using standardized tests. There is danger in placing too much reliance upon the IQ numbers without reading the psychologist's discussion of the results; there may have been unusual circumstances such as tiredness or recent testing which would affect the child's performance. Tests only sample a child's problem-solving behaviour; they cannot indicate potential in some magical way. Furthermore, a child's IQ can vary within about 15 points during maturation so that absolute stability over time would not be expected.

Modes of thinking

Preschool children think differently from adults. This is particularly important when asking or explaining reasons for things (like illness). They are likely to display the following:

Egocentric thinking (I'm tired, therefore it's getting dark). The child places himself at the centre of the world. This does not mean he sees himself as all-powerful. If things go wrong (parents falling ill), he is likely to believe that it is because of him; something he has done or failed to do. **Events are interconnected** and **all actions have a purpose** (a marble rolls downhill because it is going home). People and things **exist for a purpose** (the moon comes out at night to make it less dark; aunts exist to give you Christmas presents). According to **animistic beliefs** inanimate things and animals can behave like people (a car hurts itself in a crash). In general, there is an intuitive, magical quality to thought rather than a logical approach. It is important not to overstate the case. For instance, small children are not entirely self-centred and can empathize. What is described is a tendency to drop into such styles of thought rather than rigid constraints.

Primary school-age children are less egocentric and more logical in their approach and are particularly adept at **classification and categorization** (although they may have difficulty in realizing that an object can have more than one characteristic at a time). They tend to be **rule-bound and rigid** having to think in terms of the here-and-now. Metaphors are not easily grasped and need careful explanation.

Only in mid-adolescence does it become possible for a child to think in an adult manner, using abstract concepts, metaphors, and being able to compare various hypotheses. Doctors are good at such thinking and so it is paradoxically difficult for them to communicate with young children who do not have such cognitive abilities and who are likely to resort to replying 'Don't know' to well-meant enquiries.

Language acquisition

By his third birthday, the child can usually join at least three words and many children are using sentences of four or five words or even longer. Comprehension is normally more advanced than speech production and many 3-year-olds can understand quite complex instructions, involving three or four information words (e.g. put baby's shoes in the cupboard in the kitchen). Almost all 3-year-olds can recognize and pick out on request one of a dozen or more objects.

Articulation, vocabulary and grammar sometimes develop at surprisingly different rates. The ability to produce all the sounds of the native language is usually acquired within the first 3 or 4 years, although a few sounds may present particular difficulty and may not be perfected until 7 or 8 years of age. Some children may speak very clearly yet have a poor vocabulary or very immature use of grammar. Others may have a great deal to say, using a wide range of words and grammatical structures, yet because of poor articulation are almost unintelligible.

During the phase of very rapid language and vocabulary acquisition, many children copy whatever is said to them, as if mentally replaying a word or phrase out loud, helping them to understand better. This is called echolalia. It is a normal finding up to 3 or 3½ years of age, but if it persists much beyond this or if the child repeats words yet shows no sign of understanding their meaning, there may be some difficulty with the overall comprehension of language.

In the normal course of language acquisition, over-generalization is common, i.e. the child applies a word to all objects in a class. For example, all fruits are bananas, all animals are dogs. Grammatical rules are also treated like this, resulting in words such as 'sheeps', 'hurteded', etc. He then refines these rules and learns the various exceptions.

By the age of 4, the average child has almost mastered his native language except for some sophisticated grammatical constructions. Of course, he still needs to enlarge his vocabulary. There may still be a number of errors in pronunciation but the great majority of his speech is intelligible. He can recount experiences, listen to a short story and tell it back to the reader.

Play

In the third year of life, the child acquires various other skills such as building models or structures with bricks or Lego, using a pencil (although rarely able to draw anything recognizable much before the age of 3), doing simple puzzles, playing games with rules, etc. Attention and concentration mature and play becomes more complex with routines and sequences and an increased ability to pretend, so that, for instance, a box can represent a car or a ship.

The child's ability to concentrate on a task and to accept suggestions while playing gives some insight into the way he is likely to respond in the classroom. If the child has not reached this level of mature concentration at the age when school entry is approaching, he may not benefit from the routines of ordinary school and some special provision may be needed.

By the age of 4, he can build recognizable models and draw pictures with at least some semblance of shape and form. Given adequate opportunity, it is not uncommon for him to be able to count, read some words and write his name.

Independence and self-help

With increasing emotional security the 3-year-old child can separate from his parents for increasing periods of time, for instance to attend nursery or playgroup. He becomes more socially confident and able to cope with strange situations. Increasing understanding of daily routines coupled with greater motor coordination enable him to acquire increasing independence in daily activities such as using the lavatory, washing hands, etc., and he can assist with household tasks.

The 4-year-old has acquired considerable social poise and confidence although this may still crumble very quickly when faced with new situations. Given the opportunity, motor skill has advanced to the point where he may have learned to pedal a tricycle, catch a ball, swim, play the violin or ski! (Figure 10.1).

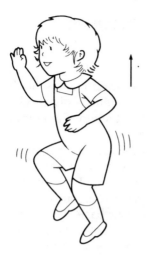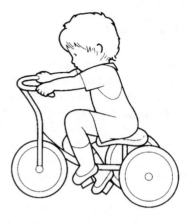

Figure 10.1. Motor skills in a 4-year-old.

Summary of the preschool review between 3 and 5 years

- Review:
    - Progress and development.
    - Behavioural and emotional concerns.
    - Growth and physical health.
- Observe and discuss:
    - Motor ability.
    - Language and ability to communicate.
    - Social maturity; ability to cope with unfamiliar situations.
- Physical examination:
    - General check.
    - Heart.
    - Testes.
    - Back.
- Measure and plot height.
- Ask if parent has any concerns about vision or hearing; check for any high risk factors.
- Carry out any specified vision and hearing checks.
- Health education topics.
- Preschool immunization.

Procedure for the preschool review between 3 and 5 years

Many Health Authorities have discontinued the traditional school entrant physical examination. Instead, the school doctor examines only those children who are causing concern to parent or teacher. It is therefore important for all children to have a check before they reach school age.

This 'school readiness check' may be done by the GP alone or shared with the health visitor. The GP should carry out a physical examination; and the parents should be given the opportunity to raise any anxieties they have about developmental progress or behaviour. The check can easily be carried out at the same time as the preschool booster is given, or on an opportunistic basis.

In this age group, the question which is often uppermost in the parents' minds is, 'How will the child respond to the new demands of school?' If they feel that his progress is slower than that of other children, they may be anxious to ensure that appropriate assessment and intervention are arranged.

It is the responsibility of the Health Authority to inform the Education Authority if there is any suggestion that the child may have special educational needs, having first discussed this with the parent. Remember that doctors can only *suggest* that the child may need an educational assessment or specialized education—it is not a medical decision.

By far the most common problem requiring differential diagnosis between the second birthday and school entry is a delay in language acquisition. This may be accompanied by more general learning difficulties of mild or moderate severity, impaired social relationships or concentration and behavioural problems.

It would be unusual for a child to present so late with an inability to walk, but other motor problems may need evaluation, for instance excessive weakness, fatigue or clumsiness.

Clinical evaluation

This consists of informal observation, history, developmental review, and physical examination.

- **Observe** all aspects of the child's behaviour from the moment you introduce yourself to the parent.
- Offer the child a few toys, then ignore him while you talk to the parent.
- Give the child the option of sitting on the parent's lap or at a small table—the latter is encouraged.
- Do not ask the child questions which require an answer until he has relaxed.
- Review **language development**, and if you think it is seriously delayed, refer for further assessment.
- Evaluate **gross motor functions**.
- Refer for **vision testing** if any concerns.
- Carry out a **physical examination**.
- Measure and plot **height**.
- Discuss the findings and interpretation, then arrange further investigations and follow-up as indicated.

- Some districts may include a routine screening test of hearing and/or vision in their procedure for this age group.

History

Review briefly the general and developmental history. If you suspect a problem in any aspect of either development or behaviour, you can *either* interview the parent for more detailed information *or* offer a referral.

Common worries include growth, appetite, sleep, colds, ear infections, chest infections. Ask the parent if the child ever wheezes; this is an easy 'screening test' for asthma.

Motor functions. Ask whether there are any worries about the child's walking. Can he run? Is there any limp or asymmetry? Can he tackle stairs? Does he tire unusually easily compared to other children?

Communication. Often the child's responses to remarks or questions from the parent within the first few minutes of a consultation are sufficient to assure you that language development is normal. If this does not happen, ask the parent if the child is talking well and if there seems to be any doubt, either refer the child or review the matter in more detail (p. 230).

There are no easy screening tests for slow language development. By the time the child is 3, most parents will already have asked for expert advice, but occasionally problems may be detected for the first time by an alert GP or health visitor.

Hearing. It is logical to ask about hearing at the same time as comprehension. For example:

- Are you sure that he can hear? Why are you sure?
- Can you speak to him from another room and know that he will understand.
- Does he respond to quiet sounds, for instance opening a biscuit packet?
- Are there any factors that might increase the risk of a hearing problem, such as family history of middle ear disease?

Concentration, attention and separation. Consider the child's ability to **stay on one task** without being distracted. Can he **play with other children** and stick to the rules of a game? Are the parents worried that he is **hyperactive**? If so, what do they mean by this term? By the time a child reaches the age of 3, parents are beginning to think about school and the child whose concentration is poor may cause them great worry.

Is he able to **separate** from the parents without becoming unduly distressed? Some shyness and anxiety in a strange situation is of course perfectly normal, but if it is excessive it may become a real problem for both child and parent, and you may feel that more expert advice is needed (p. 234).

A useful question is: **How do you think he's going to cope at school?** If there is any concern, consult with the community paediatric service or the Child Development Centre. They will arrange further assessment and will liaise with the Education Authority if necessary.

Vision. **Ask** the parent: **'Have you any worries about the child's vision?'** These are more likely to be related to squint or to a family history of amblyopia or hypermetropia as most serious defects have been detected before this age. If there is any concern, refer to the orthoptist or eye clinic. Optometrists may be willing to examine young children.

In some districts a community orthoptist (p. 67) screens children in this age group. Screening of *all* children is rarely feasible and is probably not cost-effective, but screening of children in local authority day nurseries may be worthwhile; these are often children from deprived backgrounds and although they are not necessarily more likely to have vision defects, they are less likely to receive diagnosis and treatment.

There is still controversy about the value of preschool vision screening. Do not embark on vision screening unless it is a policy of your district; in that case, insist on a demonstration of the approved equipment, and clear guidance on referral criteria. See p. 225 for a description of the method.

All children are offered a visual acuity check when they start school.

Behavioural disorders and emotional problems. These are very common. Ask whether the parents have any such worries and if so whether they can cope or whether they need advice.

Health, growth and immunizations. Ask if there are any worries regarding these and if the immunization schedule is up to date.

Examination

Language and hearing

Try to confirm the parent's description of the child's language development, by observing the child's response to the parent when they talk to him. If you can satisfy yourself that the child has normal or above-average language development, you know that he is unlikely to have any serious hearing difficulty and that he is almost certainly within the normal range of intelligence. Conversely, if there is any doubt about language or there are any risk factors for hearing loss, further assessment is needed.

A speech discrimination test using toys (McCormick Test) can be used as a way of detecting hearing loss in this age group (*see* p. 221). Ask your audiologist or community child health doctor to demonstrate this. It is easy in principle, yet even experts make mistakes because deaf children are amazingly adept at passing hearing tests!

Gross motor skills

Observation of the child's walking, running and climbing is often sufficient to exclude any disease specifically affecting the motor system.

Physical examination and measurements

The yield of routine physical examination at this age is very small, but a full examination should include:

- Inspection of the **skin** (check for unusual marks, e.g. multiple café-au-lait patches suggestive of neurofibromatosis).
- Listen to the **heart**.
- Listen to the **lungs** for wheezing.
- Check the descent of the **testes**. If in doubt about their descent, refer. If both testes were *definitely* descended at birth and at 6 weeks, it is extremely

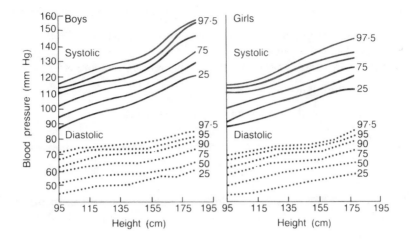

Figure 10.2. Relation of blood pressure to height in children. Figures are percentages of boys and girls. Reproduced with the kind permission of the *British Medical Journal*.

unlikely that they will re-ascend. This is why a careful check in infancy is vital and why a record must be made.
- Inspect the **spine** for evidence of dysraphism as described on p. 134.
- Measure and plot the **height**.
- Opinions differ on **blood pressure (BP)** screening in young children, but most authorities do *not* recommend it. However, the BP should be measured in children who have a history of renal disease, or growth problems. This will usually be done at specialist clinics.

  Do *not* measure the BP in children unless you have a selection of cuffs of various sizes. This is essential, otherwise substantial errors are inevitable. The cuff *must* be wide enough. The correct width is two-thirds of the distance between the shoulder and elbow. In practice, this means the largest cuff that comfortably fits around the arm (Figure 10.2).

Innocent murmurs are characterized by absence of any other symptoms or signs of disease in the CVS; often soft and musical sound; lack of radiation to back or widely across praecordium; changes with position. *Very* common; most children have a functional murmur if you listen carefully and particularly if the child is ill. Parents usually notice that you can hear something in the heart because you tend to frown and listen for longer! It is advisable to explain the concept of an innocent murmur, which is a normal noise made by the blood flowing through the heart and lungs.

Do not recall the child for repeat examinations. One re-check is enough; it will not get any easier to decide! Either make up your mind that the murmur is innocent, or refer. Even a cardiologist can have difficulty with some murmurs. Parents can become very anxious if left in doubt about a possible heart complaint; they may restrict the child's activities and worry excessively over trivial ailments.

Summary—simple rules about speech and language problems
Speech production (expressive language)
A child needs further assessment if at the age of 3 he/she is:

- Unintelligible to the family.

- Unable to produce a sentence of *four syllables*.

If at the age of 4 he is unable to:

- Be understood by strangers.

- Recount the theme of a picture.

The child may be slow in learning to speak or in **learning to understand** (*comprehension*). Further assessment is needed if he/she does not understand:

- Single words at 15–18 months.

- Short instructions at 2 (e.g. get your coat).

- Longer instructions at 3 (e.g. get your coat and take it to daddy).

A child who does not *understand* speech may be:

- Severely or partially deaf.

- Generally backward.

- Autistic.

- Dysphasic (suffering from specific language impairment).

Interpretation

If there are any concerns about language development, overall learning ability, lack of ability to concentrate, etc. the child needs a more detailed assessment (p. 230). Some children seem to speak quite clearly, but have difficulty with the **social rules** of conversation. This type of problem is difficult to recognize, but there is a strange quality about the child's behaviour and means of communication. Parents and teachers may feel that there is something wrong but not know what it is. If presented with such a story, refer for speech therapy opinion or for full Child Development Centre assessment.

Clumsy children. So-called clumsiness is a problem of motor coordination which usually presents in the early school years. The child may have problems with gross motor activities (running, riding a bike, catching a ball) or with fine co-ordination (most often with handwriting). It is not usually a disease but probably represents the bottom end of the distribution curve for motor talents. The child needs to be examined to exclude neurological disease. Management is aimed at helping his specific problems, i.e. it is education and therapy-oriented, rather than medical.

Some so-called clumsy children have other learning difficulties as well. Recently it has become fashionable to call them **dyspraxic**, but this term is still

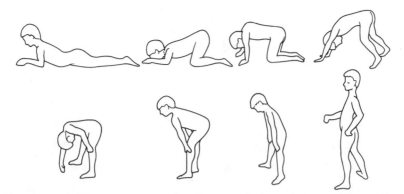

Figure 10.3. Gower's manoeuvre can be used to check for the muscle weakness which is typical of muscular dystrophy. Ask the child to lie supine and then get up. To rise from supine, the child turns into the prone position, and walks the hands up the thighs. (Courtesy of Dubowitz.)

only a description, not a diagnosis, and there is no simple treatment. Refer any such children for full assessment at a Child Development Centre.

Whenever there is concern about weakness, excessive number of falls, difficulty on stairs, etc., in an otherwise healthy boy, it is vital to exclude **Duchenne muscular dystrophy** (Figure 10.3). All that is needed is one blood test for CPK (creatine phosphokinase).

Is he dyslexic? Concerns about reading, writing and spelling usually surface in the 6–9 year age group, but occasionally parents become anxious that the child may be dyslexic even before he goes to school. This is particularly likely to occur if there is a strong family history of dyslexic-type learning problems.

It may be tempting to dismiss such anxieties as being typical of over-zealous, neurotic middle class parents; but they turn out to be correct too often for comfort. Expert assessment of such children may not be easily available either in the Health Service or in the Education Authority, but the community paediatrician or Child Development Centre may be able to help. The parents may also find it useful to contact the Dyslexia Institute, 133 Gresham Road, Staines, Middlesex TW18 2AJ. Telephone: 01784 463851.

Hearing assessment

Some districts may require all preschool children to have a hearing test, using one or more of the methods described here. Selective referral to a second-tier clinic is preferable, selection being based on criteria such as parental concern, language delay, behavioural problems, or middle ear disease.

Clinical approach

This consists of:
- History.
- Observation of child's behaviour and language.

- Co-operative tests.
- Otoscopy.
- Impedance measurement (second-tier clinic).
- Referral and treatment.

History

Ask the parent these questions:

- What do you think about his hearing?
- Why do you think he can/cannot hear? Can he for example:
  - Listen to conversation.
  - Hear key in door.
  - Hear biscuit packet being opened.
  - Hear aircraft before parent?

(Note that all these sounds are mixed frequency and the ability to hear them does not exclude a hearing loss affecting only part of the frequency range.)

- Does he respond better if:
  - You point.
  - You raise your voice.
  - You let him see your face while you speak?
- Does he say 'eh', 'what', 'pardon'?
- Do you often feel that he is ignoring you?
- Does he like the TV turned up loud?

Co-operative tests

As the child matures, distraction tests become increasingly difficult. Between the ages of 1 and 2½ or 3, testing is particularly challenging. As soon as possible, more precise tests should be substituted, using methods that require the child to make some form of voluntary response to a stimulus.

The two most popular approaches are the speech discrimination test and the so-called performance tests. A bright child will try to co-operate with these methods as young as 24 months, and over 90 per cent can be tested successfully by 39 months of age.

Test procedures

Co-operation is needed and it is important to be flexible in handling the test procedure.

The **first aim is to exclude serious problems by three tests** which can often be accomplished very quickly:

- **Simple, quietly spoken sentences** (*not* whispered) at 1 metre from child: the speaker should hide the mouth behind the hand to prevent the child from lipreading. Ask 'Where did you put your teddy?' or a similar casual question. The ability to comprehend simple questions confirms not only functional (though not necessarily normal) hearing, but also gives information about language development.

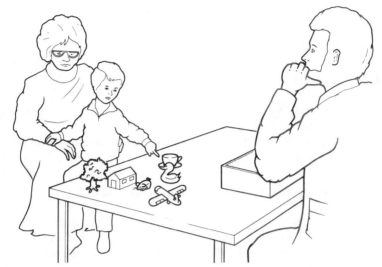

Figure 10.4. A speech discrimination test of hearing.

- Make a **high pitched sound** (rattle, 'sss' sound, warble) as described for the distraction test, when the opportunity arises.
- Check the ability to **locate a small bell or other noisemaker** at 1.5 metres from the child; this helps to rule out serious unilateral loss.

Speech discrimination tests

The ability to discriminate between similar speech sounds provides a valuable although indirect measure of hearing. The technique is easily learnt and is capable of detecting even quite minor degrees of hearing loss.

The most convenient test for screening preschool children is the McCormick toy test (Figure 10.4). This consists of fourteen toys, each with a single syllable name. The toys are paired so that they sound similar; for example, plane and plate, shoe and spoon. Very young or immature children may have difficulty with the small toys, but can sometimes be tested, albeit rather less accurately, using four or five large common objects (cup, spoon, shoe, fish, sock).

The child should preferably be seated comfortably at a small table. The test is best conducted with the examiner sitting at the table opposite the child. For screening purposes, no attempt is made to test each ear separately and one accepts that a mild unilateral loss may be missed; this will be detected at the school entry test, at the time when it becomes potentially more significant.

The toys are produced one by one and the examiner says 'here's a . . . shoe', etc., pausing long enough for the child to start naming them himself if he is willing, but he should not be urged to speak if he does not want to. The whole test can be completed successfully without the child saying a word. The parent should be asked to indicate if any object is unfamiliar. Some objects have two possible names, e.g. lamb or sheep, and it is important to establish which the child uses.

If the child's home language is not English, it is sometimes still possible to do this test, by teaching the parent to request the objects. However, many parents have difficulty in dropping the voice to a low enough level.

The examiner then says, using a normal voice intensity, 'Where's the . . .' or 'Show me the . . .'. It is essential that the child understands the game before any attempt is made to test the hearing. Once the child knows what is wanted, the mouth is covered with a hand (a bright child with even a mild hearing loss will learn to lipread without any tuition), and the voice intensity is lowered progressively with each item. Be careful not to look at the toy you are about to request as the child may follow your glance and select correctly! Make sure you do not choose the toys in any logical order.

Children of this age are sometimes rather easily distracted so it may be necessary to gently hold the child's hand and say 'Listen' several times, until you are sure you have his attention. If you think the child can understand you can say, 'I'm going to ask you to show me the toys and I'm going to speak very quietly so you must listen'.

You should reduce the voice intensity until the parent, who should be seated about 3 metres way, cannot hear what is said. This corresponds to a sound level measurement of less than 45 dB. A child with normal hearing will still be able to identify the toys correctly when this point is reached. It is surprisingly difficult to speak clearly at such low intensities, and a sound level meter is valuable as a check. The child with more mature attention control can perform this test with the tester at 3 metres distance.

A whisper should *not* be used because it lacks the low pitched laryngeal component and is therefore a higher pitched sound; in SOM the hearing loss is maximal in the low frequencies, and the diagnosis may be missed if a whisper is used instead of minimal voice.

The child with a hearing loss

After testing a few children it is quite easy to recognize the child who can only respond reliably when the voice intensity is raised, and one can even roughly quantify the hearing loss with this technique. If there is a moderate or severe hearing loss, the child may be quite unable to perform the test, yet give the impression of wanting to please the examiner, and will touch the toy immediately if the examiner points at it. The child with a modest or fluctuant loss can usually perform the task adequately when the voice level is raised a little, perhaps to the level of quiet normal speech. Mild problems in speech discrimination revealed by this test may be the only sign of SOM but may still be significant to the child.

When the level is too low for him to hear easily he may become uncooperative or anxious, turning to the parent for reassurance. Alternatively, he may try to peer behind the examiner's hand to try to lipread. Most children will join in this game quite happily and if the child does not do so it is safer to assume there is some problem than to label him as uncooperative.

Around 90–95 per cent of children aged 39 months can perform a McCormick toy test, so if a child of this age is unable to carry out the task adequately, other possible explanations must be considered. These include global backwardness, a more specific impairment of language development, autism or even a visual defect. Indeed, although the test is not intended as a language screen, it is often more than adequate to confirm that progress in this field is within normal limits.

Performance tests

Hearing may also be checked by means of performance tests. These require the child to make some form of response to a sound signal, usually involving a toy. For example, placing a brick in a basket or a wooden man in a boat. Performance tests are particularly useful when the child has difficulty in coping with a speech test, either because of limited language abilities or because his first language is not English. They also provide a useful way of confirming a hearing loss suggested by the results of the speech discrimination test.

The sound stimulus can be either voice or an electronically generated signal produced by a portable audiometer. The latter method is, of course, more precise and rather surprisingly some children seem to respond better to these artificial sounds. A portable audiometer is, however, rather expensive for routine use in primary care clinics.

Put the bricks or the peg men boat on the table and have another box beside them. Put all the bricks or men in the box. Say to the child, 'When I say "go" I want you to put the men in the boat (brick in the box).' Demonstrate a couple of times and if necessary let the parent do it as well. Most children will be eager to try themselves. Continue to say 'go' a few more times, quite loudly, to be sure that the child has grasped the idea. Then gradually reduce your voice level to 45 or 40 dB (measured if possible). 'Go' is a low frequency sound; the test is repeated using the high frequency sound 'ssss'.

Most 3-year-olds can perform this test, but at 30 months many will have difficulty in waiting for the 'go' and will become immersed in putting the items in the box or boat. This limits the accuracy of the test although you may still be able to make observations about their hearing.

It is difficult to avoid giving visual clues when doing this test and you may find you are nodding your head or raising your eyebrows while saying 'go'. It is advisable to cover your face completely with a piece of card.

Using the free-field portable audiometer, it is usual to start at 1 kHz, at 65 dB and then reduce the intensity in 10 or 20 dB steps to 35 dB. Then check all frequencies at this intensity and finally, if the child's concentration is maintained, check at 25 dB and even at 15 dB if the room is sufficiently quiet. The aim is to establish the **quietest sound that the child can hear**. Be careful that the child does not get into a regular rhythm of putting the bricks in the box; it is important to vary the interval between each stimulus. Do not give any visual clues. Even the movement of the tendon of your thumb may be perceived by an observant deaf child!

The pure-tone audiometer is not only useful in its own right but is also good training to prepare the child for a complete audiogram, using headphones. This is important because it is the only reliable way of detecting monaural losses, which although of little importance for language acquisition, may be significant at school.

Around a half to three-quarters of children in the age range 2½–3 years will learn these tasks quickly and easily. They may accept the headset of a standard pure-tone audiometer and can even do a bone conduction audiogram. Others aged 3½ or even 4 years require a good deal of time and patience to obtain reliable results.

In areas where there are many children of ethnic minorities who do not speak English, performance tests may be the only way of assessing hearing.

Otoscopy

Otoscopy is often very difficult in young children and the drum is often partially obscured by wax. Furthermore, the physical signs of SOM may be very subtle. The decision to refer a child is usually based on a history suggestive of a middle ear disorder, or on the presence of a hearing loss, rather than otoscopic findings.

Secretory otitis media (SOM) (also called otitis with effusion, glue ear) is very common in children. The most frequent complaint is of hearing loss, but there may also be pain, and sometimes a disturbance of balance. Most children have a single attack, or repeated attacks with complete resolution between each episode; but a few have severe persistent SOM and it seems likely that these may suffer a significant impairment of language development.

The **hearing loss** is typically of modest degree and fluctuates from day to day and gets worse with colds. The parent may think the child is stubborn or disobedient and may also complain that the child turns the television up too loud.

The **signs to look for are:** loss of the normal grey gunmetal sheen, with its light reflex (though this can be preserved in some cases), a blue, amber or inflamed appearance, retraction indicated by change of the normal angle of the malleus, and in suppurative otitis media, perforation and a discharge (in chronic cases, the odour may help you to distinguish between a discharge of wax and a true purulent discharge).

Treatment of SOM is controversial. There is no doubt that myringotomy and grommet insertion brings about a dramatic improvement in some children, but this is often short-lived, and at follow-up the eardrum is often thinned and scarred. Although surgeons differ widely in their views, the trend is now towards a more conservative approach, with surgery reserved for children with intractable problems. Adenoidectomy may also contribute to an improvement in middle ear function and in other upper respiratory symptoms, although it does not apparently make much difference to the hearing.

Decongestants do not help and have subtle but unpleasant side-effects. Antibiotics given for 2–3 weeks many be beneficial in some cases although this also is far from certain. Some audiologists favour the use of a low-power hearing aid, until the hearing recovers spontaneously.

Remember that SOM is very common, and may coexist with sensorineural hearing loss, so make sure that the child's hearing is retested after surgery. Particularly in the first 18 months of life, it can be very difficult to decide whether a hearing loss is entirely due to SOM or has an additional sensorineural component. Parents are often all too willing to believe that an operation will solve the problem of hearing loss and fail to attend for a post-operative hearing test.

Wax

Never attribute a hearing loss to wax until you have removed the wax using Cerumol, Otosporin (if there is otitis externa), a Jobson Horne probe, or syringing, and have shown that the hearing then returns to normal.

Vision tests

Serious congenital vision disorders have usually been detected long before the age of 3. The main aim of vision screening in this age group is to detect squint, refractive errors and amblyopia. Of these, amblyopia is the most important (p. 64). Colour vision defects do not cause significant disability in the preschool or early school years.

Districts vary in their policy regarding preschool vision screening. Some may require a check for squint (p. 63). Others only specify a test of visual acuity, while yet others have suspended preschool vision screening altogether, and make no attempt to detect these defects until the child starts school.

Clinical evaluation

History

Ask all parents:

- Have you any worries about his vision?
- Have you ever noticed a squint?

Ask the following as well if the parent is worried:

- Does he hold objects very close to his eyes?
- Can he recognize you at a distance (e.g. when you collect him from the nursery)?
- Does he feel for objects rather than look for them?
- Does he have particular problems seeing in poor light?

Visual acuity tests

The precise measurement of visual acuity requires tests which examine the ability to separate adjacent visual stimuli—the **minimum separable** tests. With these it is possible to detect the minor impairments of vision which are associated with refractive errors or amblyopia. In contrast, **minimum detectable** tests such as those using 1 mm sweets can only identify children with severe impairment of visual function.

The standard method of measuring visual acuity is the Snellen test type. The child is asked to read a series of letters displayed at a distance of 6 metres. A person with normal vision is said to have 6/6 vision.

The largest letter on the Snellen chart can be read by the person with normal vision at a distance of 60 metres. A person who could read this letter only at a distance of 6 metres would be described as having 6/60 vision. Note that this is a pseudofraction; it does not mean that the vision is one tenth of normal

The Snellen test type method of measuring visual acuity has been modified in various ways so that it can be used by young children who do not yet read letters reliably. It can be simplified by reducing the number of letters and by using a selection of letters which children seem to cope with most easily, such as V, T, O, H, X.

Children who have the opportunity to look at early reading books may be more familiar with lower case letters and one should therefore have available a lower case Snellen chart. The child does not have to be able to name the letters. A matching card can be used which can be home-made if necessary, or you can use plastic letters.

Single-letter tests

The **Stycar test** consists of five or seven letters, mounted on individual cards. Alternatively, the **Sheridan Gardener test** can be used; this has a wider range of letters of each size and because it is presented on matt rather than shiny card, it is easier for the child to identify the letters. These tests include a letter of 6/3 size. If it is essential to carry out the vision test at a distance of only 3 metres (as is often the case in primary care premises), the child must be able to read this size of letter to pass the test at a true 6/6 level.

Although single-letter tests have the merit of simplicity, they are not an ideal method of testing visual acuity because they underestimate, or even fail to identify, amblyopia. This is because of the so-called 'crowding phenomenon', which means that the child has considerable difficulty in identifying the individual letters in a line, even though he may be able to do so quite adequately when the letter is displayed on its own without distracting adjacent visual stimuli. For example, a child may appear to have 6/12 vision when tested with single letters, but 6/36 when tested with the Snellen chart.

Since the detection of amblyopia is perhaps the most important justification for preschool vision screening, single-letter tests can no longer be regarded as a satisfactory screening technique.

The **Sonksen Silver test** (Figure 10.5) has been devised to overcome these problems. It uses a line of letters with a matching card, and can be used at 3 metres. It is probably the best available test for preschool screening for visual acuity defects. However, many children lack the maturity to perform any kind of matching test and this remains the limiting factor in the screening programme and leads to many re-tests.

Whether one is using the Snellen chart or a single-letter test, it is essential to **check each eye separately**. One eye may be occluded by an eye patch with an elastic headband, or a sticky patch; alternatively, a folded tissue in the parent's hand may be used. The child should not be allowed to occlude the eye with his own hand as he will certainly peep through his fingers if the vision with the other eye is unsatisfactory. Although some very young children will tolerate occlusion at any age, many object strenuously. By the age of 39 months, most children will tolerate occlusion with a little persuasion (*see* Figure 10.5).

The test procedure

It is important to make sure the child understands the task. Seat the child at the table with the parent beside him. Set out the matching card or plastic letters on the table. Using the single-letter teaching book, teach the child the concept of matching, saying 'can you find me one like this?' As soon as he understands the task, retreat to 3 or 6 metres (you will lose rapport with many young children at the longer distance) and tell the child you are going to repeat the task.

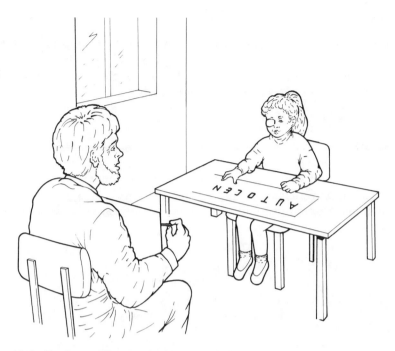

Figure 10.5. Sonksen Silver test with occluded eye.

As we have said, it is important to test each eye separately. If the child is cooperative, fix a sticky patch (Dermicel) cornerwise from the nose, after demonstrating on yourself or the parent. If he is anxious, carry out the test with both eyes open and then try again to occlude each eye in turn.

Start with the largest letter, then go quickly to the centre of the fourth and fifth lines, then to the sixth. Go back one line if the child is hesitant on the smaller letters. This procedure is adopted because the child is likely to become bored very quickly. If the child cannot cope with the line of letters, you can use the single letters (Stycar or Sheridan Gardener), but remember their limitations.

Near vision

Near vision can be measured using the reduced Snellen chart, but this is not usually necessary as part of a routine assessment of vision in the preschool child.

Referral

It is sometimes difficult to decide when to refer a child for further examination. If there is a persisting difference in visual acuity between the two eyes, amblyopia may be present and detailed examination is advisable. If the child is unable to read the 6/6 letters but can see the 6/9 size, he should be re-examined in a year's time. If the vision is 6/12 or worse in either eye and the test is thought to be reliable, the child should be referred, but if the child is still too immature to cooperate adequately, it may be preferable to repeat the test in 6–12 months.

School entrants

Every child should have a visual acuity test on commencing full-time schooling. This should be done using the Snellen chart, with a matching card if necessary. It should very rarely be necessary to make use of single-letter tests which are unsatisfactory for the reasons mentioned previously.

Television

There are a number of studies which demonstrate that there is a link between the amount of television watched by children and their level of aggressive behaviour.

Too much television appears to make children aggressive. The mechanism is obscure but there are five possibilities:

- The increase in the number of violent scenes they are exposed to, particularly when these depict real people in recognizable situations.
- The passive nature of television watching which allows fewer opportunities for developing concentration, forethought and experience in social inter-action, all qualities required in social problem-solving through skills such as sharing, postponing gratification, and negotiation.
- The amount of time taken up by watching television which reduces the opportunities for active experience. There are fewer opportunities to learn self-occupational skills.
- The amount of time parents spend watching television which can remove them from active conversation and play with their children and each other.
- Chronic tiredness from long evenings and late bedtimes.

Obviously there are times when television is a boon to a harassed parent, but the problems of excessive, inappropriate and indiscriminate watching are real.

The ideal of only allowing children to watch a small number of particular pro-grammes, chosen by them in advance in consultation with their parents, is almost impossible to achieve for some families.

Some families have the option of using a video-recorder to regulate their children's selection of programmes. Others will have to manage their children's watching by sheer discipline.

Stopping children switching the television on as soon as the parent leaves the room is difficult. One remedy is to interrupt the mains lead to the television with a 3-pin connector so that there is a length of flex with a mains plug on one end and a connector socket on the other. This can be removed by the parent and put in a drawer or pocket so that the set is inoperable. It can be reconnected when appropriate.

Common clinical problems

Assessment of children with slow development

In most cases, assessment is carried out by community or hospital paediatricians. However, a few general practitioners have a particular interest in this field and

Health education topics

- **Immunization:** preschool booster.
- **Dental care:** check diet (snacks, sweets, etc.); should have stopped bottle-feeding; check tooth brushing, dental decay, attendance at dentist.
- **Nursery, nursery school or playgroup:** child's needs for play, conversation, social learning.

  Some children are very happy to go to nursery or nursery school and separate from the parent without difficulty, but others get very upset and may take a long time to settle. Nursery nurses may suggest that the parent simply leave the child, in the belief that he will soon get used to being away from his parent. This may work but sometimes the child becomes so distressed that the parent has to withdraw the child, often with serious consequences for their job and income.

  If the parent has a child who they think might react in this way, it is probably better to accompany the child to the nursery, and stay with him; leave with him after a short period before he has a chance to get upset. Each day, the parent should try to separate very briefly from the child; at first just across the room, then outside the door for a few moments, then coming back for him after a few minutes. This may take several weeks but in the long run it will be worth it.

- Some young and inexperienced parents need to understand that their responsibility to educate the child does not end when he goes to school! Their active support and interest is vital. For example, parents can improve their child's **reading level** by listening to the child read each day.
- Management of minor ailments; e.g. admissions to hospital for wheezing can be reduced by good management and education of parents.
- Television–*see* p. 228.
- **Accident prevention:**

Age	Danger	Advice
2 years	Burns, fires	Keep matches and lighters out of reach.
	Scalds	May turn on taps, so beware of hot water. Check thermostat setting.
3 years	Road safety	Teach traffic awareness and crossing safety.
5 years	Road safety	Teach bicycle safety. Should not be on the road yet.
	Drowning	Teach principles of water safety and how to swim, if not already done.
All ages	Drowning	Reinforce previous advice regarding pools and ponds.

may wish to play a more active role in the assessment of children with problems. This section is intended to offer some guidance on the approach to slow preschool children. In the 3–5 year age group, the commonest developmental problem is concern that the child is progressing more slowly than his peers, either in language acquisition, motor co-ordination or in all aspects of development.

What does 'slow' mean?

In some developmental disorders, for instance autism or profound mental handicap, the pattern of behaviour and function is qualitatively different from that of the normal child. No-one would use the term 'slow' for such children. 'Slowness' is generally taken to imply that the child's pattern of development is essentially similar to that of a younger normal child.

How slow must a child be before he acquires this label? The problem has many parallels in medicine. How high is high blood pressure? How much overweight must one be to qualify as obese? It is reasonable to define slow development in terms such as 'a score on a standard developmental or psychological test that is more than 2 standard deviations below the mean'. This definition would include around 2–3 per cent of children. In practice, however, one does not only consider the child's developmental level of function; many other factors play a part in deciding whether to designate a child as slow.

Parental expectations. A child whose progress is only slightly below average may well be perceived as slow by highly educated professional parents, whose standard of normality is an IQ in the superior range. Such parents are sometimes described in rather disparaging terms such as pressurizing or over-ambitious but their concerns are perfectly legitimate. In contrast, a child of below average ability may be regarded as normal by parents whose own education and intelligence are limited. It is the mismatch between their expectations and the child's actual ability and temperament which causes anxiety and disappointment to the parents.

Availability of resources. All children benefit from stimulation and good teaching. The designation of the slowest 3 per cent of children as slow is no more logical than selecting the slowest 5, 10 or even 20 per cent. In reality, it is the availability of resources which determines how many children are referred for therapy or education.

Quality of parental care. Slow development can sometimes be attributed to inadequate stimulation in the home environment. Some children are less vulnerable than others to adverse circumstances and their development may remain within normal limits, in spite of an impoverished home life. Nevertheless, they may well be performing far below their true genetic potential. It follows that simply measuring the level of development can never indicate whether intervention is desirable.

The conceptual difficulty. Doctors tend to regard children with slow development as having a medical problem, which they call developmental delay. This pathology model is not shared by other disciplines. For instance, the

Much of the material in the above section has been adapted from an article by Dr David Hall that appeared in *Archives of Disease in Childhood*.

educationalist recognizes that all children need education and that some may at various times need additional specialized help in order to learn. The linguist and the psychologist are interested in the process of language acquisition, variations in development and external influences on learning. To the sociologist, slowness in children might be a reflection of poverty, deprivation and economic injustice.

Doctors should recognize that there is no monopoly of wisdom in these matters. The uniquely medical role is to diagnose those specific conditions which can adversely affect a child's development, while accepting that in most cases the diagnosis of slow development is inevitably imprecise.

Differential diagnosis

For all the reasons discussed above, it is not possible to define slow language development precisely. It becomes a problem when someone is worried.

The ability to communicate is prized in our competitive society and slowness in language acquisition is rightly regarded as an important problem. It may be a sign of some more serious underlying condition and is associated with an increased risk of educational problems in the future.

The problem presented by the parents is nearly always related to impaired production of speech, i.e. the expressive language. It cannot be overemphasized, however, that the child's ability to comprehend is equally important.

It is helpful to divide the diagnostic process into five stages:

- **What exactly is wrong with the child's speech?** The parents' account of expressive language can nearly always be trusted, and in fact they often underestimate the child's output because of reluctance to credit him with a word if the articulation is unclear. Parents worry most often about a lack of clarity in the child's speech. As a rough guide, a child's speech should be comprehensible to the family by the age of 3.

  From the prognostic point of view, isolated articulation difficulties are in fact rarely serious. More worrying is the child whose speech output is severely limited and who makes little effort to communicate. Inability to relate the theme of a simple picture at age 4 has been shown to be a warning sign of learning difficulties in primary school.

  There are a number of uncommon disorders which cause serious problems in speech production, in spite of normal comprehension, intellect and hearing. Diagnosis is difficult, but useful clues include persistent dribbling, or problems with chewing and swallowing; expressionless face; severely restricted range of individual sounds; lack of progress over a period of time; motor disorders (e.g. Duchenne muscular dystrophy and ataxic cerebral palsy can present with speech disorders).

- **Is there any impairment of comprehension?** The usual answer to the question 'How much does he understand when you talk to him?' is 'Everything'. Parents tend to overestimate comprehension, because children are good at recognizing gestures and situational clues, such as preparations for meals or bedtime. It follows that if the parents have recognized the child's difficulty in understanding, it is almost certain that comprehension is seriously impaired.

- **What do the parents feel about the child's hearing?**

- **Does the child perform normally in other respects?** For instance in play, self-help (washing, dressing, helping in the home). These are all activities which do not require language and can be learned by use of visual observation alone. A psychologist would designate these tasks as 'non-verbal abilities'.
- **Are the attention, concentration and social competence normal?** Does the child show attachment to the parents and respond normally to strangers?

Causes of impaired comprehension

A significant difficulty in comprehension is associated with four possible diagnoses, all of them potentially serious:

- If expressive language and comprehension are limited, but all other functions are normal, the diagnosis is **hearing loss** until proved otherwise. The deaf child of normal intelligence can make sense of the world through the visual channel alone. The diagnosis is still missed because both parents and doctors find it hard to believe that a deaf child can look and behave normally in all other respects.
- There are some children who in spite of normal non-verbal intelligence and good hearing, fail to develop language normally. Opinions differ on the prevalence and precise definition of this group of developmental problems, which are collectively known as **language disorders**.

Questions about what the child says

- How much does he say?
- How many single words can *you* understand? (You may find it helpful to prompt the parent—is it two or three, 10, 20 or 50 or too many to count?)
- Are there a lot of words which cannot be understood even by those who know him well?
- Does he put two or three words together to make a little sentence, such as, 'Daddy gone'? Can you give an example? (Some children learn whole phrases like 'go to sleep', but phrases generated by the child himself are better evidence of progress in language acquisition.)
- What length of sentence can he produce?
- How well does he make his meaning understood?
- Does he use words like under, on, behind, and, but?
- Can he tell you what he wants, what he's been doing; can he relate a simple story?
- Can he hold a conversation, describe something that happened, repeat a story, take a message?
- Are his words clear enough to understand? Do you understand him? Do strangers understand him?
- Are you mainly worried about *how much* he can say or is it the difficulty in *understanding* him that's the problem?

- If the child's non-verbal skills and the ability to concentrate or play constructively are also impaired, it is likely that the slow language development is a reflection of a more **global backwardness**. The IQ is usually in the borderline range of ability or just below, now designated as 'learning disabilities' rather than 'mental handicap'.

  Most children with severe mental handicap present in the first year; nevertheless, it is not unknown for a child with an IQ of 50 or less to present at the age of 36–42 months for the first time, with language deficits as the presenting feature. Usually the parents have sensed that the problem goes beyond speech development, but they seldom recognize the significance of their observations and the diagnosis of learning disability comes as a devastating blow.

Questions about comprehension—what the child understands

For **more detailed review**, you can ask parents questions such as:

- *How much* does he understand when you talk to him?
- Can you ask him to show you his nose, his feet, his eyes?
- Does he look towards familiar people when named?
- Does he understand if you ask him to do simple things, for instance to get his coat or shoes? Could he still understand if you asked him when you were in another room, so that he couldn't see you or guess what you want?
- Could you tell him to get them from a particular place, for instance could you say, 'Go and get your shoes, they're in the kitchen?'
- Would he understand more complicated sentences and ideas?
- Would he understand if you said, 'We're going out to see grandma, or to the shops in a minute and I'll buy you some sweets'?
- Does he identify/recognize colours?
- Does he know his name if someone asks him?
- Can you tell him a story? Does he follow it? Would he know if you changed the story or left something out?
- Does he frequently lose the thread of a conversation, get hold of the wrong end of the stick, get confused and go off at a tangent?

Remind the parents that children aged 3 and upwards normally understand a great deal, to the extent that parents tend to be careful what they say in front of children of this age!

It sometimes helps to ask parents to make a comparison with a younger sibling or with other children whom they know well. For example: if you said something a bit complicated, who would be more likely to understand, this child or the younger one?

This often helps parents to appreciate the extent of a comprehension problem. A 4-year-old who understands less than the 2-year-old sibling has a serious problem.

- Abnormality of social behaviour, with a lack of interest in people and failure to show normal attachment to familiar adults, may suggest a diagnosis of **autism**. The classical autistic child shows grossly abnormal behaviour and it is usually obvious that there is some serious problem. Milder degrees of social impairment cause diagnostic difficulties (*see* box below). **Asperger's syndrome** and **semantic-pragmatic disorder** are fashionable names for these often puzzling conditions.

Shy or autistic?

It may be difficult to decide whether a child is just unusually shy or has some more serious problem.

- Many young children are *extremely* shy with strangers, but they can respond normally to familiar people and most will gradually 'warm up' with people they do not know.

- Some preschool children talk at home, but will not speak in nursery or in the first year at primary school ('elective mutism'). In many of these the problem resolves spontaneously, but some also have a speech or language disorder.

- Autism is not an 'all-or-nothing' diagnosis; there is a spectrum of severity and the picture changes as the child gets older. Suspect autism if: the parents feel that the child does not relate to them in a normal way, or enjoy any form of communication, or show empathy (awareness of other people having feelings); or if the child does not pretend or play, or does so in a stereotyped repetitive way; or indulges in meaningless repetitive routines.

Differential diagnosis is not always easy: if there is no sign of improvement after a reasonable time, referral to a paediatrician, psychologist or child psychiatrist is advisable.

Clinical evaluation

History. It is important to establish who is worried and about what. If the parents themselves are worried there is seldom any difficulty with the consultation. If the suggestion that the child has a problem comes from another professional, parents may be resentful, hostile or perhaps guilty that they failed to recognize it themselves.

The value of a developmental history depends on the precision of the questions. For instance, 'Is he talking?' is vague, but 'How many words can he say, that you can understand?' is precise.

The usual information about past, family and obstetric history should be gathered. Family history is particularly important as unusual patterns of development often run in families.

Developmental examination. The way the child plays and talks, the social demeanour and response to the examination, all give insight into the child's level of maturity. It is useful to watch the child walking, and if possible running and jumping. Fine motor function can be observed by giving the child some play materials to use while the history is taken.

Look at non-verbal performance before language as it is less threatening to the child. Use bricks, crayons and paper, a puzzle or formboard, and a colour sorting task. You are more interested in the child's approach to the task than the exact level of function. One of the aims of the exercise is to decide whether the child is likely to need special help at school, so pay particular attention to concentration and ability to continue with a task. Note whether he responds to suggestions and assistance in playing. You also want to know whether there is a significant discrepancy between non-verbal and language abilities.

When assessing language, look first at comprehension. There are two reasons for this preference. Firstly, you can obtain clear information about expressive language from the parents, but they do not always find it easy to describe comprehension so precisely. Secondly, it is usually easy to test comprehension because the child does not have to give a spoken response to questions; comprehension can be tested by asking the child to respond by pointing.

Every 3-year-old should be able correctly to select one from an array of a dozen common objects when asked to do so in a clear voice. Nearly all children of this age can recognize an object by function (e.g. 'which one do you sweep with?'), and obey commands with two information carrying words (e.g. 'give the doll to mummy'). The older the child, the more comprehension he is expected to have.

The child should not be asked questions which demand a spoken response, otherwise he may simply cry or refuse cooperation. If a child does not tell you the name of a toy, tell him rather than wait for him to respond. By conveying to the child that it does not matter whether he talks, most will in fact be persuaded to do so.

Hearing and vision. This may be assessed at an audiology clinic, but ideally language and hearing should be considered together, in the same clinic. See p. 215 for details.

The possibility of a **vision** defect should be considered, particularly in children designated 'clumsy'. The child may, for instance, feel for steps with his foot before descending or bump into objects.

Physical examination. This is seldom rewarding in children with minor learning difficulties or speech and language problems. Occasionally one finds signs of a dysmorphic syndrome. A severe disorder of expressive language, or any evidence of muscle weakness, inco-ordination or spasticity, are of course indications for a complete neurological examination.

Further assessment. The doctor's role is often that of an intermediary between the parents or the professional who first voiced concern, and the multi-disciplinary team of specialists who can contribute to diagnosis. The opinion of a speech therapist is often invaluable in describing with greater expertise the nature of the child's language difficulty. A standardized test such as the **Reynell Language Scale** is particularly useful when a more precise estimate of the comprehension deficit is required. An experienced physiotherapist or occupational therapist may be very helpful in the assessment of a 'clumsy' child. A shared consultation between therapist and doctor is often an economical way of assessing developmental problems.

A formal psychometric assessment using a standardized test may be useful in children with complex language disorders or physical handicaps which impair communication. It is important to choose a test that is relevant to the question being asked. Unfortunately, most doctors are only trained to use the **Griffiths Scale**, which is not always the most appropriate choice.

Investigations

These are rarely helpful unless the neurological disorders listed above (*see* p. 218) are suspected. With these exceptions, children with speech and language problems do not need a CT scan, a metabolic workup or an EEG. The two tests which may be worthwhile are a chromosome study (Fragile-X and Klinefelter's syndrome) and a CPK to exclude Duchenne muscular dystrophy.

Formulation. In explaining the situation to the parents, try to distinguish between (a) the presenting functional problems and (b) the cause. For instance, terms like speech and language disorder and learning difficulties describe the pattern of difficulty, but give no clue to the cause. Of course, in the majority of cases we simply do not know what causes these problems. Parents like to know what they are *not* due to; brain tumours and perinatal brain damage are two common worries.

Perinatal damage related to anoxia in a full term baby should *not* be accepted as the cause of a learning or language difficulty unless there was severe neurological illness in the neonatal period, and even then it is wise to be cautious; once you have even hinted at the possibility of brain damage, the parents may become both upset and litigious. Leave any such speculation to a specialist. A family history of slow language development or general learning problems is often obtained, suggesting that genetic predisposition plays a part in many cases.

Other possible causes of developmental problems include prenatal dysmorphic syndromes and severe intrauterine malnutrition. Environmental deprivation is undoubtedly important in some cases and may be accompanied or preceded by a history of non-organic failure to thrive. This can however be a damaging and cruel diagnosis; even if parents are not actually told that their child's problem is being attributed to poor parental care, they can usually deduce that this is what the experts think.

Intervention. It is essential to find out what the parents feel about intervention. Some resent the stigma which they feel is attached to a medical label and prefer intervention to be offered in an educational rather than a medical context. In this view they are supported by the Education Act of 1981, which describes children as having special needs rather than defects or disorders.

The literature on preschool intervention suggests that:

- It is possible to help children with a variety of special needs.
- Any programme which involves parents has a greater chance of success.
- Attitude and adaptation to adult life are likely to be improved more than actual levels of performance.

Encourage parents:

- To seek and accept preschool help.
- To look at the content and quality of teaching and care being offered rather than the name of the school or unit.
- To regard therapists as consultants, who should advise the parents and teachers as well as working directly with the child.
- To recognize that the education system cannot ever replace parents.

Information for parents. The parents should be offered a written report (with their agreement a copy should be sent to the local Education Department), a leaflet about the Education Act and details of the appropriate voluntary organization(s).

What to do if parents want speech therapy advice

- The parent should visit the local health centre/community clinic and ask how an appointment can be made.
- If this is not successful, the GP or parent can write to the senior manager of speech therapy services in the Health Authority. If you have difficulty finding out who this is, call the Community Services offices, or call:

> The College of Speech and Language Therapists
> 7 Bath Place
> Rivington Street
> London EC2A 3DR
> Telephone: 0171-613 3855

Behavioural and management problems

The remainder of this chapter is concerned with common behavioural and management difficulties of preschool children and those in their first year or two at school. Effective techniques for intervention can be mastered by primary care staff and the ability to deal with these common problems will be of benefit to the practice as a whole.

The main disadvantage of the techniques described here is that parents must be properly counselled in their use and this takes time.

Success rates will improve with practice. It may therefore be sensible for one particular member of the primary care team to develop their skills in this field as an area of special personal interest. Alternatively, the practice may choose to employ a clinical psychologist on a sessional basis to deal with these problems. However, few GPs will have access to such expertise and many staff, particularly health visitors, may derive considerable satisfaction from solving these common behavioural problems themselves and from the improved relationship with the parents that follows the elimination of a troublesome behavioural problem.

Sleep problems

This is a common clinical problem of preschool children with a prevalence of about 10–20 per cent. Although apparently trivial, the stress on parents is severe, not least because they are exposed to a great deal of advice, most of it useless. Everyone seems to be an expert, but the problem persists. Although there are a multiplicity of causes, they can readily be managed according to Figure 10.6.

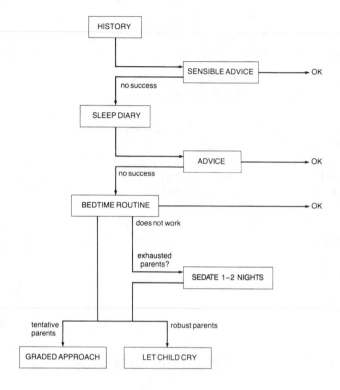

Figure 10.6. Difficulty in settling: overall management.

Difficulty in settling at night

See both parents if at all possible and tell them that:

- This is a common problem, not usually a sign of bad parenting or a spoilt child.
- It is not always easy to deal with; there are no guaranteed short cuts.
- Even adults find it difficult to fall asleep by effort of will.
- Their first duty is to survive, not to win a battle.

A small child who just will not go to sleep at the expected time may be:

- Not tired because he has had too long a sleep in the afternoon.
- Not tired because he has been over-stimulated or excited just before bed.
- Not tired because he customarily sleeps late in the morning (mother lets him sleep in because he got off to sleep late the previous night). Thus his sleep period is displaced later than usual but is of normal duration, so that he is getting an adequate amount of sleep and is not tired at the early evening bedtime.
- Frightened of being left alone or abandoned (normal separation anxiety).
- Anxious because of noises in the dark, parents having a row downstairs or because he knows he will eventually make his mother angry.
- Confused as to what is required of him (mother puts him to bed before father gets home but he knows father is pleased to see him when he gets in; different bedtimes every night, etc.).

WEEK BEGINNING	time awake	mood on waking	daytime naps (give times)	time told to go to bed	time in bed	time asleep	waking in night (give times)
Monday							
Tuesday							
Wednesday							
Thursday							
Friday							
Saturday							
Sunday							

Figure 10.7. A sleep diary.

The first step is, therefore, to obtain **a good account of the problem**. What exactly happens and why is it a problem for the parents (lack of privacy, tiredness, losing a power struggle, criticism from grandparents, lack of support from father)? You may be able to give **sensible advice**.

Next is to extend this to establish what the child's **sleep pattern** is. This may lead to giving sensible advice straightaway. However, as parental accounts are not always clear, it is sensible to ask the parent to keep a prospective **sleep diary** over the next week. This should include:

- Time awake in morning (and whether needed waking).
- Mood on waking (many parents report no ill-effects of failure to settle until the problem is resolved, whereupon they comment upon the child's improved mood).
- Times and duration of naps during day.
- What time he is told he must go to bed.
- What time he is known to be asleep.
- Whether he wakes during the night (time, duration and parental action).

Other details may be included (but can be omitted in most cases), such as:

- What time he is taken upstairs.
- Which parent takes charge.
- How they prepare him for bed (baths, stories, warnings, drinks, etc.).
- Whether/when he calls out or comes down.

The diary can be drawn up on a sheet of paper (*see* Figure 10.7) rather than in a booklet and is best kept near the child's bed. Explain to the parent what it is that you want by drawing up columns and headings or by having a prepared sheet.

This may establish something that you can give sensible **advice** about:

- Unreasonable parental expectations.
- Too much sleep during the day (think about getting him into a playgroup) but note that a *brief* early afternoon nap can improve the quality of night-time sleep.
- Erratic bedtimes.
- Displaced sleep cycle.

It is wise to **set a bedtime** (saves repeated ill-tempered negotiations each night) and establish a **bedtime ritual** with a fixed progression of events—from a warning that bedtime is approaching, through taking the child to his bedroom, undressing him, bath, tucking up, story, kissing goodnight and so on. This enables a small child who cannot tell the time to be aware of the approach of bedtime. The number of calls for glasses of milk, etc. should be limited in advance. The bedroom must be congenial and enhance falling asleep (nightlight, etc.).

The essential task is for the parent to help the child to learn how to fall asleep on his own. Either setting a bedtime and routine is sufficient or further measures are needed. If the latter, pause for thought.

If the parents are at their wits' end and exhausted, consider **medication** for the child for 1 or 2 nights. Trimeprazine tartrate as Vallergan Forte syrup in a dose of 45–60 mg about 2 hours before bedtime usually works although the child may be irritable the following morning for a few days. It may take several nights to get the dose and timing right but a maximum of 2 weeks is a good rule for sedating a small child. Make sure the parents continue to use the 5 ml plastic spoon issued: domestic teaspoons can hold as little as 1.5 ml with consequent disappointing results.

Once the parents are feeling braver discuss two options with them.

Letting the child cry. This is quick if the parents can manage it. Many parents will say they have tried it and it does not work. Closer questioning reveals that they could not stand the screams and gave up too soon.

Firstly make sure that the environment is conducive to sleep. A soft light (nightlight or landing light), toys in the bed (not exciting ones), and a tape recorder playing a story all help.

The following steps are necessary:

- Both parents must agree with each other that they are going to do it properly (no dishonour in feeling it to be too brutal).
- They *must explain* to the child what is going to happen: that once he has been kissed goodnight, they are not going to come in to him when he cries and that they want him to lie quietly in his bed and wait until he falls asleep
- The child should not be able to get out of the door but should be able to reassure himself that the parents are still around and have not deserted him. A burglar chain on the door or a stairgate in the doorway are useful ploys.
- The parents need to let the child know that they are still around. They should be urged to talk, sing, wash up noisily or have the radio or TV on. This is in contrast to the usual parental practice of creeping around silently to let him get to sleep.
- The parents must have something to do besides listening to the screams or they will not be able to stand it.

HELPING A CHILD FALL ASLEEP ALONE

HOW LONG TO WAIT BEFORE GOING IN TO CHILD (IN MINUTES)

DAY	FIRST TIME	SECOND TIME	THIRD AND SUBSEQUENT TIMES
1	5	10	15
2	10	15	20
3	15	20	25
4	20	25	30
5	25	30	35
6	30	35	40
7	35	40	45

SHUTTING THE DOOR ON A CHILD WHO GETS OUT OF BED (MINUTES)

DAY	FIRST TIME	SECOND	THIRD AND SUBSEQUENT
1	1	2	3
2	2	4	6
3	3	5	7
4	5	7	10
5	7	10	15
6	10	15	20
7	15	20	25

Figure 10.8. Helping a child fall asleep alone.

- They may also have to warn the neighbours.
- The total duration of crying before sleep should be recorded on a chart (*see* Figure 10.8).
- Both parents must understand that the crying *gets worse at first*. Like all behaviour intended to attract or be perpetuated for social attention, crying will initially intensify and last longer if attention is withdrawn. If the parents can last out for the first 4 nights, the crying should then gradually subside. The record kept will show this more clearly than the recollections of a fraught and somewhat guilty parent.
- Next morning the child can be praised for going to sleep on his own. He can stick a star on a chart or a bead on a string at the foot of his bed.

Managing things gradually. This graded approach takes longer but is more acceptable to many parents. The core programme is as follows but may require some preparatory work if the situation is out of hand (*see* p. 242).

Again parents agree the procedure, tell the child, have a contingency plan for when the child screams.

- Parent (mother for the sake of illustration) settles child briefly, *without letting him fall asleep* and leaves the room, telling him she will return in 5 minutes. The bedroom door is left ajar.

- She does not return for 5 minutes unless the child gets out of bed in which case she returns him and tells him that she will shut the bedroom door if he gets out of bed again.
- After 5 minutes she returns to the child and settles him briefly (about 2 minutes) and then leaves the room *before he falls asleep.*
- 10 minutes later she returns and settles him briefly again.
- 15 minutes later she visits again and subsequently visits at 15 minute intervals until the child is asleep. She must always leave the room before the child falls asleep since the object of the exercise is to help the child to learn how to fall asleep on his own. All she has to do is quieten him.
- Getting out of bed after the first warning is dealt with by the mother taking the child back to bed then going out of the door and holding it closed for a full minute. She can talk through the door to the child, telling him that if he goes back to bed, he can have the door left open. This can be repeated as often as necessary, increasing gradually the time the door is held closed (*see* Figure 10.8). Talking through the door is allowed. Once he has returned to bed, at least 5 minutes should elapse before the parent returns to settle him.
- After the first night, the time intervals are subsequently increased by 5 minutes each night, i.e. for the second night, 10 minutes to the first settle, then 15, then 20 (*see* Figure 10.8). Similarly, if the child gets out of bed, then the time that the door is held shut is lengthened progressively.

Most children will be settling well by the end of a week. Nearly always, the problem has resolved before reaching 45 minute timings.

Preparatory work. Some parents will have virtually lost control of the situation and be spending enormous amounts of time in the child's bedroom. If the child is used to a parent sitting by (or lying on) the bed or cot, start from there. Get the parents to take alternate nights on duty to share the burden. They must stop lying on the bed next to their child and move to sitting on the edge, then, over a number of evenings, to a chair by the bed, then moving the chair each evening nearer the door until eventually they are outside the door. They should have something to do other than watch the child: reading, knitting, crosswords, even listening to a personal stereo. If they have been singing the child to sleep for hours, get them to hum increasingly softly each evening. The principle is **very gradual change**.

Some children, mainly the 3-year-olds and over, can be encouraged by a simple **incentive scheme**. A string tied to the bed or hung next to it can be used to store large beads or buttons earned for completing certain tasks. These must start with the possible, for instance the child getting into bed himself once he is dressed in pyjamas. When that has been established for a week, a new task is set and different colour beads are earned for the next stage such as lying down while a story is read, then a new colour for lying quietly while mother goes downstairs for 3 minutes, and so on, each stage worked upon until it has been established for at least a week. It can, of course, be used in conjunction with the graded approach programme outlined above.

If the problem is coming out of the bedroom once well settled, the child can be rewarded for coming no further than the top of the stairs, then to the bedroom doorway, then for doing that without calling out and so forth. The ultimate aim is to have the child lying peacefully in bed, prepared for sleep, and staying there for an adequate amount of time.

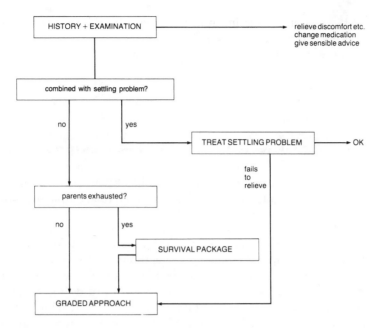

Figure 10.9. Waking at night: overall management.

Helping the child to fall asleep without a parent in the room is the aim of the exercise.

Waking at night

Most small children wake during the night but only some make a fuss about it. There tends to be an association with settling difficulties because the child who cannot get to sleep in the evening without a parent present will have the same difficulty when he wakes in the night. In such a case **treat the evening settling difficulty first**. A variant of this is that the child may be able to fall asleep at bedtime with the landing light on, the television easily heard and the traffic outside. In the middle of the night it is dark and silent. It may therefore be a good idea to duplicate these conditions at bedtime (no lights, no noise from downstairs, etc.).

The child who settles comfortably in the evening yet wakes and cries in his own room (or comes into his parents' room) at night should be examined to exclude a physical cause for discomfort: eczema, asthma, otitis media, glue ear (often overlooked as a cause of night time discomfort), teething, etc. The possibility of medication (especially bronchodilators) as a cause of insomnia should be reviewed. Other obvious problems such as noisy neighbours (or parents) or recent stress may enable sensible advice to be given. (*See* Figure 10.9 on management.)

Some parents of frequent wakers will be too exhausted and the nights too cold to implement a treatment programme straightaway. For such reasons the following advice (**survival package**) seems realistic as a medium-term measure (several weeks):

- Parents agree to take alternate nights on duty (saves the arguments and point-scoring about whose turn it is); the child cannot insist upon the other parent dealing with him.

- If initial attempts to soothe the child or return him fail, then the parents can be given licence to take him into their bed.
- The parent not on duty moves out into any spare room or bed available for the rest of the night.
- If the child manages to stay in his own bed throughout the night without crying he is praised accordingly in the morning. He can earn stars for being found in his own bed in the morning.
- Medication (trimeprazine 60 mg at bedtime) can be added to take the edge off things but should only be used as a short-term measure (1–2 weeks) to allow parents to overcome their own sleep deprivation. Earlier studies which suggested it was ineffective have been overtaken by the demonstration that a dose of 45–60 mg provides a reasonable (although not complete) respite.

The risks of taking a small child into the parents' bed have been exaggerated. It is an extremely common practice and in most instances has no long-term sequelae. Taking the child into the parents' bed at the beginning of the night is a different matter because it interferes with their sex life, but this argument does not necessarily hold for the child who is taken in or allowed in during the night. Parents fear (or are told) that they will never get him out again but in real life this does not seem to be a problem, particularly if the child is constantly reminded that staying all night in one's own bed is a sign of growing up. The cost is that the child will never learn to get back to sleep alone in the night but it may be sensible to postpone having to teach him how to if the nights are cold.

The orthodox advice for managing children who come into their parents' bed at night is to return them straightaway and wait outside the door, calmly returning them to bed each time they emerge. However, this is arduous as it may have to be repeated twenty or thirty times a night.

Therefore, parents who are ready to deal more definitively with the problem of a waking or wandering child should apply the **graded approach programme** (p. 241) in the section on settling difficulties, complete with the door-closing sanction. They return the child or go in to him and settle him briefly, returning after an initial 5 minute period, lengthening this gradually. It may be wise for the parents to arrange a strict alternate nights rota to avoid arguments.

A child who wakes early (4.00–6.00 am) is difficult to manage. Sedation often will not work. If he wanders alone around the house at such a time and thereby puts himself at risk, then the best that can be done is to ensure that there is an adequate supply of toys in his room and keep him there with a stairgate in the doorway. If the problem is that he comes in to the parents too early, tell them to put a time-switch on a bedside nightlight. If set for an appropriate time in the morning it provides the child with a visual indicator of when it is appropriate to come in to the parents. This can be linked with returning him if it is too early and, conversely, praise (perhaps with stars on a chart) for not disturbing them.

Nightmares and night terrors

Nightmares are bad dreams and occur during REM sleep. The child may cry out or wake, in which case he is clearly frightened and clingy. The contents of the dream can usually be recalled at the time or in the morning. Nightmares are common, particularly between the ages of 5 and 10 years and do not require any attention unless they are more frequent than once a week (as a rough rule) or unless there is a strong repetitive theme to the content, indicating a morbid preoccupation. It is possible to suppress them with a tricyclic antidepressant such as amitriptyline or clomipramine (not trimipramine which does not suppress REM sleep) but hardly ever necessary to do so. Generally speaking, preoccupations frightening enough to dominate ordinary dream content and produce essentially the same nightmare over a period of weeks merit psychiatric referral.

The exception is recurrent nightmares following an identifiable traumatic experience such as an assault or serious accident, in which case combine amitriptyline 50 mg at night for 1 month with attempts during the day to get the child to talk to a parent or a trusted adult about the incident in question, and to play imaginative games or draw pictures related to it. Some theories of the mind claim that dreams, as well as reflecting daytime experiences, assist their accommodation into memory, raising the question as to whether it is sensible to suppress dreams with medication. Formal studies of REM deprivation do not demonstrate any harm arising from dream suppression and, whilst it is wise not to meddle unnecessarily with sleep, a short course of a tricyclic antidepressant can free the child from avoidable terror.

Night-terrors are an instance of so-called parasomnias (*see* p. 246) which arise out of one of the first phases of very deep (stage 4) non-REM sleep, in other words before midnight and often about 1–3 hours after falling asleep. The parents hear a loud shriek or loud burst of crying and run to the child who is found sitting up in bed or stumbling around the bedroom with open eyes. They may notice a racing pulse, dilated pupils and terror: signs of a very high level of psychophysiological arousal. The child may appear hallucinated, fending off invisible attackers with his hands, and may call out briefly to them. He will push his parents away and not cling to them. It is impossible to get through to him in spite of his appearing awake. After a few minutes he returns to sleep and has no memory of the episode in the morning.

Such attacks are much more common than most textbooks imply although no formal prevalence figures have been established. They seem to be particularly likely in children under 5 although they can occur at any age. It used to be said that they indicated deep psychological disturbance but there is no evidence for this in preschool children, although their frequency will increase if the child is stressed. Nor is there any justification for the assertion that they reflect a disturbance in their parents' sex life, although given the timing of a typical night-terror, it can certainly disrupt it. The myth persists because the sex life of many parents of young children is likely to be at a somewhat unsatisfactory stage in any case, for a number of understandable reasons.

The appropriate course to take with night-terrors is:

- To **reassure** the parents. They should be told that the phenomenon is a disturbance of sleep which the child will grow out of. They should not try to wake the child during a terror.
- To keep a prospective record of recurrent night-terrors so as to identify the time at which they are most likely to occur. Once this is established, the parents should **fully wake the child 15 minutes before the projected time** each night for a week, subsequently allowing him to go back to sleep after 2–3 minutes (anticipatory waking). This often abolishes the problem by

encouraging the development of a different pattern of sleep stages. It can often, with good effect, be extended to the treatment of other parasomnias (see below).

In the unusual instance of excessive frequency (e.g. more than one night in three for 1 month) of resistance to the above method, night-terrors can be abolished with diazepam 2–6 mg at bedtime since benzodiazepines inhibit stage 4 sleep. Although it might seem logical to use a short-acting benzodiazepine, this can merely postpone the terror until the final hours of the child's sleep which is even more disruptive to parents' sleep. Continue for 3 weeks, then discontinue gradually.

Sleep-talking, sleep-walking, thrashing in bed and tooth grinding

Normal preschool children are likely to show brief movements such as face rubbing, squirming, muttering or moaning, and abrupt sitting up in bed about 1–2 hours after settling. These occur for a few seconds as the child emerges sharply from the first phase of very deep (stage 4) sleep. If pronounced or prolonged they are called **parasomnias**, phenomena arising out of a disturbance in the integration of the stages of sleep and not a result of disturbing dreams. They are typical of older, mainly school-age, children and are all common. Usually there is a family history. They can be listed on a scale of increasing severity from brief, unsettled episodes as described above, to dashing around the house in confused panic.

Sleep-talking rarely requires medical intervention beyond reassurance. It can be suppressed by anticipatory waking (if regular in its timing) or a benzo-diazepine, but this is hardly ever necessary.

Sleep-walking is potentially dangerous; there is no truth in the adage that sleep-walkers come to no harm. The parents must ensure that the bedroom windows are secure and consider putting a gate across the child's doorway. It may be wise to move the child to the lower bunk bed where this applies. Older children may manage to reach the front or back door and these will then have to be locked or bolted with a high bolt.

There is no point in waking a sleep-walking child; they will have no memory of the episode in the morning. Although obviously confused whilst walking, they are not basically psychologically disturbed and the best course of action is nearly always to steer them back to bed gently and play the whole thing down, ensuring that the child is safe. If there is a regular pattern, waking the child 15 minutes before a likely episode each night for a week, as for night-terrors, will usually work. If absolutely necessary benzodiazepine suppression (diazepam 2–5 mg at bedtime for 3 months) can be implemented. This may be necessary if the disorientated sleep-walking child is prone to urinate in cupboards, or if night-terrors and sleep-walking combine so that the child rushes around the house in confused panic. Even so, it is wise to obtain a prospective record in case a pattern can be established and anticipatory waking tried first.

Some children **thrash** around in bed in a confused, inaccessible state which may occasionally go on for several minutes. They lack the apparent fear of a night-terror but usually respond to a week of anticipatory waking.

Tooth grinding in sleep (bruxism) seems likely also to be a parasomnia. The usual empirical remedy, however, is dothiepin 50–75 mg at night rather than a benzodiazepine. If severe and protracted, a dental opinion may be necessary to check for enamel damage.

Night rocking, banging and head rolling

A number of small children develop rhythmic habits which seem to help them get off to sleep. These include sitting up and rocking backwards and forwards or side-to-side. They are harmless, even when quite alarming head-banging is involved, and nearly all children have abandoned the practice by the age of 4. The appropriate intervention is reassurance and practical measures to minimize noise (padding cot sides, putting foam under the cot legs). It may occasionally be possible to set a metronome to match the frequency of rocking and then gradually slow it, night by night, starting it off as the child settles to sleep.

Growing pains

Typically the child wakes at night with severe pains, usually in the lower leg. After 20 minutes or so, with parental attention and rubbing the affected area, the child settles back to sleep. The cause is not known, but the pains seem to be entirely benign. The parent may consult the GP because of unspoken fears about malignant disease (leukaemia, bone cancer).

Investigation or referral are only necessary if:

- The pains are not in the legs.
- The pain is always localized to one spot.
- The pain is prominent during day-time activity.
- There are other symptoms or positive physical signs.

Hyperactivity

In general parlance, the term 'hyperactive' is imprecise. It may just mean a high level of motor activity or can include over-activity together with a short attention span, excitability or impetuousness (this is the technically correct use). It may be used variously to indicate a symptom, a syndrome or a disorder.

Many parents describe their child as 'hyperactive' without this necessarily meaning that he is, in fact, pathologically overactive. He may thus be:

- Normally active for his age but his mother may, in her turn, be: a novice parent and does not realize the high activity level of young children; chronically tired; of a quieter temperament than he is or depressed.
- Active at the wrong times such as meals and bedtime, or in the wrong places such as shops or the back of the car.
- Disobedient—not sitting still when told.
- Not overactive but impulsive, noisy, uninhibited or distractible, qualities which affect the *style* of his behaviour.

This indicates the need for a good descriptive and developmental history, possibly with a home visit to observe the child on his own territory. A number of children can be boisterous at home or in a playgroup yet compliant and contained in a surgery or clinic. Check mother's mental state, particularly for depression which can make her an ineffective controller of children's exuberance, may alter her judgement so that she perceives a normally active child as overactive, and can induce provocative, high-amplitude behaviour on the child's part—he has to do more to obtain a response from her.

This initial assessment may suggest that:

- The child is not overactive but there is a handling/behavioural problem with noisy non-compliance or abusiveness.
- The child is somewhat overactive and has not enough to do which is quiet and absorbing while extending his capacity to concentrate (often as a result of too much television).
- The child is overactive and has parents with inappropriate expectations of self-restrained behaviour.
- The child is overactive and has a parent who is depressed.

These problems need relevant advice or intervention. Bear in mind that the child may not be entirely normal; he may have an excitable, extroverted temperament.

Some overactive children are **developmentally delayed**; their activity is commensurate with their mental age rather than their chronological age.

Overactivity can be **iatrogenic**: benzodiazepines (especially clonazepam), phenobarbitone, promethazine and metoclopramide have all been implicated as causes of inattentive restlessness.

Dietary constituents are often blamed, yet there is no evidence that they are common causes of overactivity (*see also* p. 29). Many parents will experiment with diets themselves. A tiny few succeed; the GP will see the failures. GPs should be wary of trying dietary manoeuvres without the advice of a dietician; malnutrition is a real risk. Remember that diets are expensive.

Once the above have been excluded, there are three main causes of serious overactivity, usually associated with inattentiveness in children:

- **Anxiety** in those children who respond to their anxious mood by nervous overactivity. They may have multiple phobias or a history of a recent life-threatening event. There will be a history of recent acute onset rather than a story of overactivity 'since day one'. They should be considered for counselling on an individual or family basis and referred to a department of child psychiatry if there is no progress after a few weeks.
- **Pervasive hyperactivity (hyperkinetic disorder)** in which the child is, and always has been, overactive, restless and inattentive in *all* situations and is never still unless asleep. Many (but not all) have delayed development and some degree of mental handicap. It is often said that they are brain-damaged but there is no association between brain damage and hyperactivity. The condition is rare and requires referral to a developmental paediatrician or child psychiatrist for a full neurological, psychological and educational assessment and consideration of medication (stimulants or haloperidol) or behavioural therapy.
- **Situational hyperactivity** in which the child is overactive in some situations (particularly the classroom) but not in others, and may appear quite normal when first seen. This is a common problem, especially among boys, and often associated with such traits as impulsiveness, excitability, distractibility and fidgetiness. A considerable number are also naughty or even seriously anti-social. Not surprisingly, educational problems are frequent and may require an assessment by an educational psychologist.

Situational hyperactives are a heterogeneous group. Their overactivity will often respond to stimulative medication but this is difficult to handle without

2 to 5 years **249**

experience and is essentially palliative. A sensible first line of approach would be to advise the parents to:

- Adjust their expectations according to the child's capacity (e.g. shorten the duration of meals).
- Provide structured, sedentary activities (puzzles, drawing, models, Lego) and actively encourage the child to carry them out by himself. Note that allowing the child to run around to burn off excess energy does not work except *in extremis* when the child is ultimately too exhausted to do anything at all.
- Reward such sedentary self-occupational activity by praise.
- Respond to noisy outbursts calmly and firmly.
- Maintain or build poor self-esteem by finding behaviours or achievements to praise.

Failure of such measures should lead to referral to a child psychiatry service or a developmental paediatrician.

Aggressive behaviour

(*See also* **Tantrums**, p. 204).
It is usually sensible to think about aggression as a quality of behaviour rather than a drive or a trait in its own right which the child has too much of. This helps avoid silly suggestions such as punchbags which are intended to help the child to get it out of his system (but do not work).

The causes of aggression are multiple, but the following points may be useful to remember:

- Aggressive responses are likely to occur when a child feels threatened or **provoked** beyond self-restraint. A child who is repeatedly thwarted, taunted, hit or demeaned by parents, siblings or peers can strike back.
- Aggressive responses can be **learned**. A child may learn from the example provided by aggressive parents, whether angry, brutal or harsh. Aggressive acts may enable a child to get his own way or snatch toys, thus obtaining rewards for such a style of behaviour.
- There is a close link between aggression and **mood**, particularly anger, resentment, tension and irritability. A child in a bad mood is likely to behave aggressively.
- Aggressive responses are essentially **primitive** and are likely to be deployed when the child knows of no other response which will suffice. This means they are more common among younger children and those who have learned no other way of coping with provocation.
- Aggression is a remarkably **stable** characteristic of behaviour. Once established as a general way of coping, it does not usually go away; reassurance that it will subside with time is likely to be wrong.

Not uncommonly several of these factors underlie the clinical problem of an excessively aggressive child. Families which are bad at teaching alternatives to aggression (such as self-restraint or negotiation) also tend to teach children how or when to be aggressive by using aggression to solve problems in personal relationships (employing harsh physical punishments, having rows, making physical or verbal threats). Aggression therefore arises out of a mixture of learning unacceptable responses and a failure to learn acceptable ones.

Given a parental complaint about a child's aggressive behaviour, the first obligation is to review the general status of the child:

- **Mental age**. Is there any learning difficulty or any other impairment to learning more civilized behaviour?
- **General mood of the child**. For example, is the problem essentially one of unhappiness?
- **State of the family**. Justified hatred of a preferred sibling; teasing; expectation of a new step-mother to be loved; irritable and depressed parent?
- **Sources of failure or sensitivity** with friends or at school.
- **Physiological**. Chronic pain or fatigue. Check **hearing** in a toddler.
- **Pharmacological status**. Benzodiazepines (sometimes given to the child by the parents from their own supply), some anticonvulsants.

A straightforward remedy may become apparent.

Secondly, it is important to understand how a typical episode occurs through carrying out an **ABC** analysis (p. 76). This may reveal unreasonable and unrecognized provocation in the eyes of the child, what constitutes aggression in the eyes of the parent, and how it may be being aggravated by the consequences.

This will often indicate some areas of weakness which can be remedied by straightforward advice or action. Should matters appear less clear-cut, the following are necessary:

- Arrange to see both parents and persuade them that aggression indicates a **deficiency state**; something is missing because alternative and more mature ways of coping have not been learned sufficiently well.
- When their child does behave aggressively, they must tell the child that he is doing so and that it is unacceptable (**labelling**) using a sharp, brief interjection such as 'No—I won't have that'. (This must emphatically *not* become a nag or conversational commentary on the child's actions such as 'You really ought to stop doing that . . . it's not at all nice to other little boys; they won't like you . . . .') They must tell him what he could be doing which is acceptable (**identifying desired alternatives**).
- They should be encouraged to set up a **star chart** or other incentive scheme whereby the desired alternatives (pro-social actions which supplant aggressive responses) can be encouraged.
- Suggest that they demonstrate through their own actions and interactions how problems between people can be resolved without aggression.

Failure of such an approach to yield results within several weeks is an indication for adding **time-out** (*see* p. 264). If this fails to improve matters, make a referral to the department of child psychiatry or psychology earlier rather than later.

Aggressive behaviour in the playground

A child may be aggressive because he considers it a sensible way to solve an interpersonal problem (whether or not he knows of any other way) or because he is too angry or upset to deploy more considered tactics such as negotiation.

A complaint that a small child hits, pokes or bites other children, apparently without provocation, should therefore lead to **questions about the child**: can he participate in verbal (rather than non-verbal) exchanges? Does he know of other methods of resolving disputes and can he learn these? Impaired hearing and global learning disability need to be ruled out accordingly. A few children with secretory otitis media will intermittently have sufficiently impaired hearing to misinterpret what is said to them and react to what they wrongly perceive as hostile overtures from peers.

It is important to enquire about **the child's home life**. Do the parents habitually resolve their difficulties with him or each other by aggressive coercion or violence so that he has learned the wrong lessons? If not the parents, what about older siblings? Some children are upset and angry because of insecurities or injustices in their home life.

Advise carers to **intervene immediately** at any outburst of aggressive behaviour. Place the child in a corner (observed but isolated from social interaction) for 5 minutes and, when he is receptive, describe to him more appropriate ways of behaving along the lines of 'What we do here is . . .'. Often this comes down to basic skills of sharing, turn taking, asking nicely, and doing simple deals ('If you let me . . . then I'll let you . . .'). Moral remonstration along the lines of 'What would you think if someone did that to you?' or 'What if everyone did that?' are doomed to failure as the preschool child cannot readily enter into that sort of hypothetical reasoning.

Helping the victim not to cry may be important. Patterson's classical study in a playgroup demonstrated that aggressive, coercive behaviours between young children are rapidly learned and that tearfulness when victimized provokes further aggressive attacks by others. There are a few small children, usually with impaired empathic skills, who have a malicious interest in causing pain to others because they are fascinated by their overt distress or helpless fury. Even for them the appropriate first line of management is supervision, prompt intervention for safety's sake, and tuition in alternative, civilized ways of managing disagreement or conflict.

Eating problems

Meal refusal

A preschool child is brought in by his mother with the complaint that he will not eat; mealtimes have become a battleground. At a casual glance the child is well nourished and healthy.

The first thing to do is **obtain a good account of what happens at a typical meal**. This may reveal:

- Meals irregularly timed, no constant pattern.
- Unsuitable or unacceptable food (for some children, fish, potatoes or green vegetables are genuinely nauseating).
- Multiple opportunities for distraction (people coming and going, television, etc.).
- Unreasonably large portions.

Next, ask **what the parent is most concerned about**. This commonly reveals concerns about:

- Nutrition.
- Discipline.

The issue of nutrition can nearly always be dealt with in an entirely straight forward way by weighing and measuring the child and referring to a growth chart, discussing the result with the parent.

As far as discipline is concerned, first ask the parent whether they remember being upset by foods as a child, and what other people (particularly grandparents) have said about the child's eating and behaviour at meals. This helps place things in perspective.

Thirdly, ask **how much the child eats between meals**. The initial answer is often 'nothing much', but persist. The child is getting food from somewhere.

Any doubt over these issues should lead to a request that the parent complete a **food diary** for several days. All food eaten (including sweets, crisps and biscuits) is to be entered, as well as the food that is refused. If the child's eating goes in phases, continue long enough to get an overall picture. This usually enables you to make some commonsense observations.

As a first move: **absolutely no eating between meals**. No sweets as rewards, no snacks and care with high calorie drinks. This is where parents *can* control things (in the last analysis they cannot force a child to eat). Warn parents about buying foods that they do not want their children to eat. Note that some foods are invisible to some parents who apparently do not regard crisps, sweets or chocolate as food.

A variation on the theme is that the child does eat plenty of what the parents regard as junk food—baked beans, chocolate and crisps—but he will not eat 'healthy' foods. The weight chart will confirm your statement that although it would be nice to persuade the child to eat a 'healthier' diet, he will certainly not fade away; beans, chocolate and crisps provide fat, carbohydrate and protein!

Only then move to giving advice about meals themselves.

If a parent chooses mealtimes as the arena where discipline is to be imposed they are likely to be unsuccessful. Nothing can coerce a stubborn child to eat except hunger. It is a battle no parent can win.

In general terms take the pressure off the child and the parent:

- Offer the child less to eat than usual.
- Do not rush the child (within limits; there must be an end to the meal).
- If he refuses a particular food, take it away and offer an alternative.
- No nagging, coaxing, threatening, or blackmail, no urging 'one more mouthful'.
- No fuss about the order of courses, finger feeding or strange tastes and practices. They can be put right later.
- Involve the child in food preparation.
- Avoid too many drinks during the meal.
- Encourage anything which will defuse tension at mealtimes and make them more fun.

It is usually helpful for the parent(s) to eat at the same time as the child, re-inventing the concept of a family meal. This gives him the opportunity to learn how to behave at mealtimes through observation.

Pica

Pica is the habit of **eating substances not normally regarded as food**. It should be distinguished from mouthing of objects, which is a transient developmental phase (*see* p. 196); if mouthing is still occurring beyond the age of 2 it is likely to be associated with some developmental problem such as general backwardness.

Toddlers sometimes experiment with eating undesirable substances such as dog faeces or Plasticine. During this usually brief phase of development it is very important that dangerous materials are kept locked away, and parents should check their garden for poisonous plants such as laburnum.

Parents are most likely to seek advice in an emergency because the child has eaten a potentially hazardous substance. A poison centre may be contacted for information. Remember that while repulsive items like faeces rarely seem to do any harm, some apparently innocuous substances may be deadly, e.g. crystals from a chemical set can be highly poisonous.

If the child persists in eating non-food substances and there has been no response to normal disciplinary approaches, consider the following:

- The child may have some developmental disorder. If there is any evidence of backwardness or retardation of language development, consider referral to a developmental paediatrician.
- There is an association between pica and iron deficiency. The precise nature of this link is uncertain but a short course of iron can do no harm and is occasionally very effective.
- If the child is eating *very old* paint or other potentially lead-containing substances, consider whether a blood lead estimation should be done. (Lead pencils do not contain lead.)

  Older children, usually boys, may acquire a dare-devil reputation by accepting challenges to eat increasingly repulsive items like slugs. The activity is quite difficult to eliminate and such reputations once acquired are guarded jealously. Serious harm is unlikely to result. The child may need some help in devising acceptable ways of declining these challenges without losing face.

Bedwetting

All children wet the bed in infancy; progressively fewer do with advancing age. There is no absolute, fixed age at which ordinary bedwetting becomes the pathological condition of nocturnal enuresis, so the two terms are used interchangeably here. Clinicians vary as to when they routinely actively treat bedwetting. Many would do so from age 7 but if there is substantial distress and family concern, children as young as 4 can be managed effectively. The argument for not treating early as a routine is firstly that a (rather small) proportion of 4-year-olds and over will spontaneously acquire dryness and secondly because 4- and 5-year-olds can be frightened by the sound of an enuresis alarm in the dark.

Relationship to developmental delay

Most enuretics seem to have an **isolated developmental delay** in acquiring nocturnal bladder control. In such cases there are no clues as to causation beyond a family history of enuresis (which may not be obtainable unless both parents are interviewed). It is not uncommon for children with enuresis to have one or two other instances of specific developmental delay (speech, motor co-ordination, etc.).

Mental handicap is an obvious cause of delayed acquisition of nocturnal bladder control.

Relationship to psychological disturbance and stress

Most enuretics are psychological healthy; only about 20 per cent are psychologically disturbed and in a number of children this is quite likely to be the consequence of bedwetting rather than its cause. The usual assumption is that secondary enuresis (that with an onset after a period of dryness) is most likely to relate to stress events or psychological disturbance. This is a generalization and only partly true. Primary enuretics can be disturbed and secondary enuretics not so.

In most instances of enuresis there is no clear association with recent stress. Nevertheless, bedwetting *can* occur as a response to acute stress such as bereavement or starting a new school and in such circumstances it is usually time-limited and does not commonly present as a clinical problem. If it does, provided that the stressor is clear-cut and the onset is within the last month, it can be treated expectantly. More commonly there is **chronic stress** (such as an acrimonious parental relationship) and this is likely to reflect a more complex mechanism; the source of stress may also have interfered with the normal acquisition of dryness. In such cases it makes sense to treat the enuresis symptomatically as a first move, not to try and remove the stress since this is almost certainly a protracted process if it succeeds at all.

Physical causes

Urinary tract infection. A small proportion of enuretics have demonstrable bacteriuria. Treatment of this may relieve the enuresis.

Faecal soiling associated with faecal retention is commonly associated with enuresis, presumably in part because of a distortion of pelvic anatomy and consequent restriction of bladder volume and dysfunction of the basal plate and neck of the bladder.

Polyuria secondary to diabetes (mellitus or insipidus) or renal failure can exceptionally present as enuresis (nearly always with polydipsia and often associated daytime wetting).

Anatomical causes of enuresis are extremely rare:

- An ectopic ureter opening into the vagina in girls.
- A neurogenic bladder.

Both cause continual dribbling by day and night rather than bedwetting alone.

Epileptic seizures could theoretically cause enuresis but, in practice, enuresis is no more common among children with seizures.

It follows that assessment of the enuretic child will include a history and examination to rule out the above aetiological factors, even though most cases will not have an identifiable aetiology. It is wise to include a brief interview with the child which may reveal sources of stress unknown to the parent, indicate whether the child is suffering from a depressed mood, and document the child's own reaction to his bedwetting.

Management

History

- Duration and course with relationship to obvious life events.
- Associated daytime wetting?
- Excessive thirst—sufficient to wake child for drinks at night?
- Dysuria?
- Associated soiling?
- General level of development.
- Associated emotional and behavioural problems?
- Family history of enuresis?
- Who sleeps where?
- Past and present methods of dealing with it.
- Attitude of child to wet beds?
- Attitude of parent to child and to wet beds?

Examination. This is unlikely to reveal anything, but indicates that the problem is being taken seriously. General inspection of abdomen and back to exclude palpable bladder and spina bifida occulta or other spinal lesion. Examination of genitalia.

Examination/testing of mid-stream urine

- Sugar.
- Proteinuria, many white cells, evidence of chronic renal damage—very rare.
- Infection.

Treatment

The above steps will have effectively ruled out conditions to which enuresis is secondary and the following require management in their own right:

- Mental handicap.
- Acute stress.
- Urinary tract infection.
- Faecal retention.
- Anatomical lesion.
- Diabetes (mellitus or insipidus).
- Chronic renal disease.

These can be dealt with appropriately.

Assuming that there are no clues in the history to suggest infection and a stick test reveals no excess protein or sugar, the mid-stream urine specimen can be despatched to the laboratory and the child and parent attended to.

Reassurance is the first step. The child can be told that bedwetting is quite common and that there will be at least one other person in his class at school who is bedwetting. If there is a family history of enuresis, he should be told that too. His parents should be told in his presence that it is something he cannot help.

Punitive practices should cease and the problem made easier to live with. Newspapers and a plastic sheet could go into the bed underneath the bottom sheet. Nylon sheets dry more quickly. A duvet filled with artificial fibre is more easily washed. Wet sheets are stripped in the morning and can be washed and dried so that the child has a warm, dry bed to get into each night. The child should wash in the morning rather than be sent to school smelling. Any urinary dermatitis can be treated with a barrier cream: Drapolene, Siopel, etc. Stop excessive fluid restriction in the evenings; it has no effect.

Promote social learning and self-esteem. Suggest that the parent deal with wet beds in a matter-of-fact way and meet dry beds with exaggerated approval and pleasure. There is an argument for getting them to say 'That's terrific' or 'How wonderful' rather than 'Well done', as the latter implies that the dryness is achieved by conscious effort. If the child has been creeping into the parents' bed after wetting, this should be stopped as it may function as an unintended reinforcement for wetting.

A star chart with stars for dry nights must be kept by the child and can be put on open display unless the child is embarrassed, in which case it can go inside a wardrobe door. The parents keep the stars. A common practice is to award a gold star when three consecutive dry nights are achieved. This should be continued for 4 weeks. There is no need for the parents to back the stars up with any tangible reward.

At 4 weeks, review the chart with child and parent. Show approval for successes; this pleases and motivates the child and can provide a demonstration to the parent of good praising technique. It will either show a decreasing frequency of wetting (in which case continue, reviewing at 2-week intervals) or a reasonably stable pattern which forms a baseline for the next stage.

A star chart is effective in its own right in about one-third of cases. If it is not, proceed to an **enuresis alarm** (previously known as the bell and pad). This must be given to the child as his alarm and demonstrated to him and his parents. Alarms are not available on prescription; parents can buy their own from manufacturers at a cost of about £30–40, but a better system is to keep a couple or so in the surgery, purchased by donated funds. The local department of community child health, paediatric out-patients or child psychiatric service will all have their own stock, and referral can be made to them if all else fails. It is nevertheless preferable to keep your own supply and move smoothly from star chart review to adding the alarm without loss of therapeutic momentum. Alarms can be booked out on loan.

Alarms operate on the principle that voided urine completes an electric circuit (by bridging a gap or by linking dissimilar metal pads which then act as a battery), and sounds an alarm. There are three main types of alarm:

- The alarm is the size of a matchbox and is pinned to the child's pyjama top. It contains a tiny battery and emits a penetrating buzz which may be pulsed. It connects to a small square of plastic on which are two concentric electrodes. This sensor is placed inside a perineal absorbent pad (Vespré or similar) which is, in turn, put inside the child's underpants so that it is held next to the urethral orifice.
- The alarm is a box (commonly the size of a half pound box of chocolates) which goes on a chair by the bed, just out of arm's reach. It contains a battery and emits a loud buzz. Two wires lead to two large wire-mesh or aluminium foil pads which are placed, one on top of the other in the child's bed, under the part where the child sleeps. They are separated from each other by a sheet and from the child by another sheet.

- A similar alarm connects to a single PVC pad on which are two separate, concentric adjacent metal ribbons. The pad is covered by a single sheet upon which the child sleeps.

Demonstrate the alarm to the child in his parent's presence. He is then asked to explain it himself all over again to his parent. The small alarms can be set off with a wet finger on the electrode. Demonstration of the larger alarms will involve making a mock-up on a chair using the mesh pad(s) and old sheets or kitchen paper between and over them. Sit the child on the pad(s) and pour some salted water between his legs onto the pads, triggering the alarm. In the presence of his parent show him how to turn it off and demonstrate all the ways in which he can stop the apparatus working. This lessens the chance of covert sabotage later. Give the alarm to him and think about putting his name on it with a sticky label to emphasize the point that it is his for the time being. Point out that the alarm cannot give him an electric shock. If asked, you can be reassuring as to safety. There is no risk of psychological trauma in a 7-year-old, and 'buzzer ulcers' no longer occur.

The buzz of the alarm must wake the child or it is useless. In order to ensure this, the larger alarm boxes can be fitted with a separate booster or, more simply, put in a biscuit tin. The parents will need to get up the first few times it sounds to check that the child wakes and gets out of bed when it sounds. He should go to the lavatory, then strip the bed or remove the small alarm. There is no need to reset the alarm for the rest of the night; he can go back to bed. For simplicity, two layers of bedding can be used separated by a plastic sheet which is stripped with the wet sheet.

In the morning, dry beds are rewarded by a star on the **star chart which is continued throughout the alarm treatment** as a record. The parents should telephone you after the first night to ensure all went well. Thereafter, contact should be every 2 weeks or so, preferably by appointment or home visit to see the child and praise progress. Full dryness is likely to take at least 8 weeks to achieve, maybe longer, and the child must be told this.

Unfortunately, all alarms are technically unreliable and the parents must be told to notify the surgery or clinic immediately a fault arises so that a replacement alarm can be provided. It is wise to telephone or visit the home after the first night and weekly thereafter to check the alarm is still in working order.

If the larger alarms are used the child should sleep without pyjama trousers or a long nightie. There is a small risk of excessive sweating setting off the alarm in which case cotton sheets may prove more reliable than nylon. Mesh pads usually need replacing every 4 weeks or so; once they have become lumpy they are less efficient and broken wires can penetrate sheets causing short circuits. Aluminium pads may be reduced to pulp very rapidly and are less popular than mesh. Pads made of copper braid are robust in themselves but are commonly vulnerable at the point where the wires to the alarm are connected.

It is not absolutely necessary to treat every single night, in fact there are grounds for not doing so since this cuts down the chance of relapse. Other ways of minimizing the chance of relapse include **overlearning** where by the child, once dryness has been achieved for 2 weeks, starts to drink a glass of water before going to bed. He is warned that this is likely to result in a wet bed or two but the alarm will teach his bladder to hold on to this extra load. When dryness has been re-established for a week, he is asked to drink two glasses of water at bedtime.

Once dryness has been established under this regime, the alarm and the bedtime drink are both discontinued simultaneously.

The alarm, coupled with a star chart, is a highly effective treatment provided that the child and parents are satisfactorily engaged in the process and technical faults dealt with promptly. About 1 in 5 children will relapse after dryness has been achieved, sometimes after a delay of several weeks. The alarm is reinstated until dryness is achieved. A second relapse is extremely unlikely.

Although the alarm might seem to be contraindicated in families where the enuretic child shares a bedroom, in practice the others in the room quickly learn to sleep through the buzz. Should this not occur (or if the child is deaf) a vibrator alarm can be used. However this has the disadvantage of not alerting the parents.

When there is an urgent need to establish dryness, **imipramine 25–50 mg at night** will stop bedwetting in most children. However, in nearly all studies when it has been used alone the relapse rate during the months following discontinuation of the drug has been very high and it cannot be considered an effective treatment in its own right. Most clinicians who believe that it works well use it in conjunction with a star chart which begs the question as to which is the active treatment. There is a risk of accidental overdose (especially by the enuretic child's younger siblings), it may disturb sleep, usually produces hypertension, and the anticholinergic side-effects can be unpleasant. It is best reserved for first aid measures such as staying overnight with friends or going to cub or scout camps and followed up by an alarm treatment. There is no point in combining it with an alarm.

Desmopressin, a synthetic ADH analogue, is given as a nasal spray before bedtime and may also be a sensible short-term intervention, subject to the same high relapse rate as imipramine. Similar comments apply to oxybutynin and viloxazine.

Faecal soiling

Faecal soiling, defaecation in the wrong place, is **abnormal after the age of 4** and is much more common in boys. The term **encopresis** is usually used as a synonym for soiling but is used in a more narrow sense by some people it is better to avoid it. In practice, most soilers are also constipated with a loaded rectum but this cannot be taken for granted.

Common causes of chronically loaded rectum include:

- Presence of a fissure because of pain on defaecation. Note that a fissure can follow rectal loading as well as cause it; a vicious cycle is easily established.
- Intercurrent illness with bed-rest or dehydration causing constipation.
- Fear of defaecation (punitive or anxious potty training), of sitting on the lavatory, or of using school lavatories.
- Systemic causes of constipation: hypothyroidism.
- Imipramine given for enuresis.

History

General history allows exclusion of systemic causes of constipation and assessment of development (exclude mental handicap).

- Has the child ever been continent?
- What constitutes soiling; frequency and nature of episodes.

- What have the parents done so far?
- Attitudes of the parents and child to problem.
- Associated abdominal pain, anal pain or wetting.

Examination

- Abdomen: faecal masses?
- Anus: visible fissures?
- Rectum: presence of faeces, whether hard or soft, is abnormal.

It is sometimes difficult to ascertain whether the child is constipated from the history alone since frequent soiling and urgency can result from a chronically loaded rectum.

If there is an anal fissure and no local anaesthetic is to hand, a plain abdominal X-ray will indicate the presence of rectal loading.

Investigation

Plot child's weight and height on a growth chart.

Review

Review the child's general medical history and satisfy yourself that organic causes have been excluded (hypothyroidism, Hirschsprung's disease, anal stenosis, neurological disorders, etc.) and that the child is of normal intelligence. If in doubt, specialist assessment is essential before embarking on the programme outlined here.

Management: the empty rectum

If the rectum is empty, there are five possibilities:

- The child has **never been trained**. Advise parents to institute a star chart with stars earned for defaecating in the lavatory.
- **Recent stress** (such as starting a playgroup or the birth of a sibling) has caused recently learned continence to be lost. Sympathy and a star chart usually suffice.
- **Mental handicap** with the consequence that the child has a mental age too young for continence to be acquired or the slow rate of learning has led the parents to give up trying to train him. Advise parents as to appropriate expectations and approaches.
- **Chronic diarrhoea or steatorrhoea** which episodically overwhelm the anal sphincter. The child is likely to be underweight and the stools will be abnormal. Refer to a paediatrician.
- The child is **intentionally defaecating** in a place which is chosen to offend a parent or other care-giver. The stool is well formed with a pointed end and well placed, for instance in the parent's shoe or bed. This is different from the practice involuntary soilers often adopt of trying to conceal soiled pants or their contents by tossing them under the bed or wrapping them in newspaper and putting them out of sight in a cupboard. Rather similar principles apply to smearing; some disturbed children will smear aggressively and may write insults with fingers dipped in faeces. More commonly, however, smearing of

a wall or curtains is the result of a child trying to clean his fingers after he has put them into soiled pants, or results from 'finger-painting' by a mentally handicapped young child who has just defaecated on the floor or in a nappy which has been taken off. Intentional placing or smearing is obvious, hostile, and indicates a serious problem in relationships with parents. It merits referral to a child psychiatrist.

Management: the full rectum

The commonest variant (*see* Figure 10.10). The rectum and anal canal are chronically loaded and distended so that the child loses sphincter control, has habituated to distension and no longer receives a call to stool. He may have so much loss of rectal wall tone or such hard faeces that voluntary evacuation is impossible. There may also be a problem with daytime wetting because of the distortion of pelvic anatomy secondary to acquired megacolon. Incontinence arises because of mechanical displacement of rectal contents by descending colonic contents or as a result of physical exercise. Obstruction of the rectum by hard faeces can result in liquefactive fermentation of faeces proximal to the blockage and consequent spurious diarrhoea.

The first step in treatment is to **explain** (with the aid of a diagram) to child and parent how soiling happens; the parents of a soiling child do not usually realize that he may be retaining faeces and will view the prescription of laxatives with suspicion unless their rationale is explained.

Secondly, it is imperative to **empty the child's rectum**. In most cases an oral laxative will suffice. Hard faeces will respond to a mixture of a stool softener such as docusate and an osmotic laxative such as lactulose. Soft faeces can usually be evacuated by stimulant laxatives such as sennosides although an initial daily dose of 30 mg may well be required. It is often sensible to give the dose at night to avoid crises at school. Failure to respond to oral laxatives within a week is an indication to add a micro-enema twice daily for 2 days. A phosphate enema will move virtually anything but if this also fails, refer to a paediatrician.

Once the rectum has been cleared, a **maintenance dose of laxative** should be continued in conjunction with a **diet rich in fruit and fibre**. Many children will not eat cereals with a very large content of bran because they dislike the taste so parents will often need to include baked jacket potatoes, vegetables and wholemeal bread in the child's diet.

In conjunction with this, the child will need to learn to keep his rectum empty by **defaecating in the lavatory daily**. He may be unwilling to do this at first because of anxieties he has about lavatories and defaecation but will usually respond to encouragement and sympathetic support from the parents. Children who are frightened of falling in the lavatory are often reassured by having a pile of telephone directories to rest their feet on. Those with a fissure will need local anaesthetic applied before attempting to defaecate. The child will need open access to the lavatory, particularly at times of day when he has been most likely to soil and should spend adequate time on the lavatory once there. Success in having produced a stool should be witnessed by a parent who must respond with extravagant praise and provide a reward in the form of a star on a **star chart**. Further soiling episodes are treated as accidents and noted, with minimum fuss, on the same chart, which then provides a record.

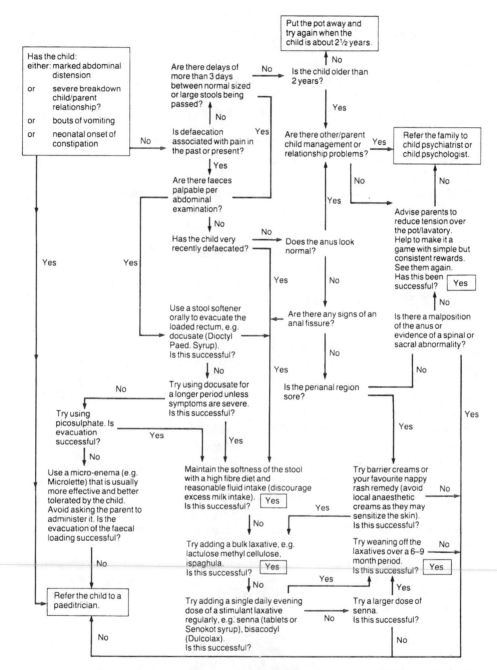

Figure 10.10. Flow chart for help available for pot refusal/constipation in children (with acknowledgements to Dr Graham Clayden).

The chart should be reviewed every 2 weeks and the programme maintained for at least 2 months, at which time the laxative can be gradually discontinued over the next few weeks whilst keeping the chart going as a record. It is difficult to maintain children's enthusiasm for star charts over such a long period of time and it may be necessary to tie in some back-up incentive such as money, bearing in mind that this can cause its own difficulties. Unfortunately, a chronically distended rectum will take months to shrink back to normal size so that protracted treatment is nearly always necessary. A return of the child's feeling that he 'wants to go' is a good sign.

It is often sensible to send an explanatory letter to the child's school doctor who can, if parental permission allows, discuss arrangements to cope with accidents at school. These may include sanction to be excused class without question, to use the staff lavatory, and to keep a clean change of clothing at school.

Failure of such a regime may occur for the following reasons:

- Rectum not completely emptied at beginning or not kept clear subsequently. It is generally held that repeated rectal examinations are not a good thing but the alternative is either ignorance or repeated abdominal X-rays.
- Instead of promoting defaecation in a lavatory, the parents have rewarded clean pants. This usually drives the child back into retention.
- The child is so apprehensive that he denies the problem to himself and will not fully cooperate. Alternatively it may be the case that he is so miserable or anxious that he just does not concentrate on his treatment programme.
- The child is so low in self-esteem or the parents are so fed up that the will to succeed is feeble. The child's school may prove unsympathetic; humiliation there can also undermine motivation.
- The soiling, although having primarily a physical basis, is also maintained by psychological factors such as secondary gain or masked protest.

Faecal soiling is a serious complaint. Everyone despises and shuns a soiler. It needs to be taken seriously and treated enthusiastically in order to maintain the motivation of the child and parents. Either party can become disastrously exasperated and demoralized. If no satisfactory regime has been established after 12 months of effort, referral is indicated, preferably to a clinic with a declared interest in this problem.

Children who are wetting as well as soiling usually become dry when the rectum has been emptied and pelvic anatomy returns to something like normality. Should this not occur, then the wetting will need investigation and treatment in its own right.

Incentive schemes

The simplest incentive scheme is the star chart but ticks on a chart, beads on strings, beans in a jar and so forth are all alternatives. Star charts have a rather dubious reputation for being impotent but, if carefully implemented, are remarkably powerful agents for promoting changes in behaviour.

Typically they are used to build compliance or otherwise get the child to do something which is already in his repertoire, but not done often enough. Perhaps because they are often effective in their simplest form, star charts in particular are likely to be applied casually. This underlies a frequently heard objection that they work at first, but the child loses interest quickly. When systematically applied, this is not a particular problem.

An advantage of star charts or ticks on a calendar over devices like beads in a jar or on a string is that they provide a written record of day-by-day achievement which may reveal whether, for example, weekends are particularly difficult. The term star chart is used here for simplicity; the principles are the same for all schemes.

To obtain maximum value from a simple points scheme such as a star chart, the following steps are crucial:

- **Establish, ideally with both parents in the presence of the child, exactly what has to be done to get a star**. Avoid being vague about goals ('be good') or attitudes and relationships ('be more helpful'); adhere to observable behaviour that everyone can recognize and agree upon. This is likely to take the form of 'If you get dressed by yourself in the morning you will get a star for your chart. You have to put on all the clothes that are put out on your chair and do up all the buttons.' The behaviour earns the point, not the manner in which it is carried out unless this can be quantified (e.g. within 1 minute of being asked). The child should, at the end of this operation, be able to specify what he has to do to get a star.
- **Agree with parents and child how the stars and chart are going to be kept**. The parents keep the stars and, when these are earned, dispense them promptly, together with praise. The chart may be displayed prominently or privately (in an exercise book or pinned inside a wardrobe door). Wherever it is, the child must be able to see it when he wants to.

  To maximize the chances of success, encourage the parents to promote conditions which make the desired behaviour more likely to occur. Frequent opportunities to learn that a desired behaviour is rewarded by a star and praise means rapid learning. There should be early opportunities to succeed; early goals should be within the child's reach and stars be frequently and promptly dispensed. When these are given to the child they should be paired with specific (pointed) praise such as 'well done for getting dressed'.
- **Clarify whether stars or points can be cashed in for tangible rewards**. It is not necessary to back up stars with rewards if the programme is to last less than 1 month. Beyond that, interest wanes and it may then be necessary to arrange for them to be exchanged later for something such as a toy, money or a privilege once a specified number of stars has been earned. The conditions for dispensing such a reward need to be agreed. Some parents want rapid results and insist on ambitious and unrealistic targets coupled with huge rewards ('a bicycle if you have no more fights with your brother'). Failure is inevitable, rapid and bitter. The general rule is small rewards, preferably privileges, dispensed immediately and contingent upon small improvements. Success is encouraged by making it as easy as possible for the child to achieve; nothing succeeds like success.
- **Examine how the scheme could go wrong**. Ask the parents what will happen if the child does what is required but grumpily; whether they will give stars for other desired but unspecified behaviour or if they are going to take stars away for subsequent bad behaviour (usually a bad idea). If stars ultimately earn money for the child, what happens to ordinary pocket money and what happens if granny gives him £5? If the programme succeeds and he earns

rewards, what about jealous siblings? If the child earns enough stars for a particular privilege within a few days, what happens for the rest of the week?
- **Specify how the programme should be reviewed**. With the above principle in mind, frequent reviews to examine how reinforcement and behaviour links are necessary. Ask the child to bring the chart in for you to see and spend some time looking at it with him.
- **Agree what constitutes ultimate success**. Parents often have a less ambitious view than clinical professionals about what a suitable conclusion of treatment should be. For instance they may want the behaviour brought under control rather than abolished. This may save time and demoralization caused by attempts to achieve 'cure' which exhaust family and child.

Such a programme is considerably more sophisticated than the simple instruction to 'put him on a star chart for good behaviour' and is vastly more durable and more effective. It is clear that a number of mechanisms underlie this apparent effectiveness. The establishment of such a programme facilitates the use of praise by parents, enhances parent–child communication, increases parental sensitivity to their child's behaviour, establishes a culture of success and so on. More than simple learning is involved.

Response cost

For some problem behaviour where it is more difficult to specify exactly what the desired behaviour is, a 'response cost' scheme may be indicated. The simplest form is to tell the child he is to be issued with a supply of points at the beginning of a time period and specify the behaviour which will lose him points. At the end of the period, points which remain can be exchanged for rewards such as food. This is only really suitable for children with some grasp of numbers and works best for short periods of time such as shopping trips or car journeys. Such schemes often go wrong, particularly because the child gets angry at being fined. There is also the problem of what happens when the child has used up all the points allocated.

Time-out

The common abbreviation for an American term '**time-out from positive social reinforcement**'. Unfortunately it is commonly misunderstood as meaning enforced confinement in a small room; which is not always the same thing at all. The principle is that behaviour, particularly bad behaviour, may be maintained by social attention which is rewarding to the child. Removal of social attention when bad behaviour is exhibited will thus, it is argued, led to the behaviour becoming less frequent. It is, in other words, a form of ignoring.

Not all behavioural problems are maintained by attention; some represent a child's attempts to preserve self-esteem or resolve tension. A history of the problem is therefore an essential preliminary. If this suggests that there is a link between the problematical behaviour and parental (or sibling) attention, then three possibilities for intervention exist:

- Encourage the parent to provide **more attention** (i.e. praise and interest) generally and especially **for desired behaviour**. It is quite often the case that

the nagging or criticism dealt out by the parent for bad behaviour is effectively the only attention available to the child.

- Discuss how the parent might **ignore** the child's bad behaviour.
- Draw up a plan whereby the child is **removed** (or told to remove himself)
  from the parent's presence when he misbehaves.

The usual course of action will be to combine one or more of the above. A star
chart is one instance of how a parent's attention may be brought to bear on
positive behaviour. It is better to structure parental behaviour by explaining
exactly what to do rather than give general exhortations to be more consistent.

Choosing between ignoring or removing the child is essentially based on
practicalities. A large child cannot easily be manhandled which may mean it is
impossible to remove him from the presence of a parent without a battle (which
would invalidate the whole procedure). Under such circumstances the parent may
have to remove herself from the room or merely turn her back and refuse to say
anything *at all* for a few minutes (structure ignoring).

Most parents will prefer to remove the child from their presence because this is
a measure which can be instituted when other people such as siblings are present,
otherwise they may pay attention to the child while the parent is ignoring him. It
is necessary to give some thought as to which might be an unstimulating place
(socially or otherwise). Bedrooms and bathrooms, although often used, may be
quite interesting places even when socially barren. The hall is, for many houses
and flats, the most boring room. Valuable fragile objects should be put somewhere
else and the front door locked as a precaution.

Setting up a time-out programme needs some planning. The child should be
told what will happen. This is based on a **1-2-3 rule**:

1. When he misbehaves he will be told to stop.
2. If he does not stop, he is warned he will have to go to time-out (or be ignored).
3. Continued misbehaviour leads to him being put into time-out (or experience
   structured ignoring).

A reasonable guide for setting the duration of time-out is **1 minute for each year
of age**. It is also important to **avoid releasing a child from time-out when he is at
the height of a tantrum**, otherwise he may learn to scream in order to obtain
release and attention. Wait until the tantrum has started to abate; it is not
absolutely necessary to wait until it has completely subsided.

A record of the number of times time-out is instituted each day, with the duration
of each episode, is valuable. Such a progress record can demonstrate several things:

- An **extinction burst**. Following the withdrawal of attention, any behaviour
  which is maintained by attention will initially worsen as if the child is striving
  to regain the attention which has been lost. The usual duration of this is only
  a few days but it is the commonest reason for parents giving up ('it made him
  worse'). Warn them beforehand and welcome it if it starts to happen; it is
  a sign that time-out will work because it indicates that the behaviour is
  responsive to attention.
- The child's behaviour may be improving (fewer episodes of time-out) even
  though he is not contrite or apologetic when released. Time-out need not be a
  weapon in a power game to be effective; tell parents not to expect contrition
  at first. If the child blusters ('I don't care; I like it'), they should take no notice.

It is not meant to be a maximally aversive punishment but a treatment intervention which needs to be repeated many times. It does not work instantaneously.

- The child may be spending too much time in time-out so that he is being generally starved of opportunities for involvement and positive family attention. He will then continue to misbehave in order to stimulate involvement, even when this is negative.

Failure of a time-out programme indicates the need to reconsider:

- Is the child misbehaving due to such reasons as emotional confusion or communication breakdown, which need sorting out first?
- Is he misbehaving because he lacks the knowledge or skills to act more positively (fights with sister because he has not learnt to take turns)?
- Is time-out really **time-out from social reinforcement**?

INDEX